Pedagogies of Biomedical Science

This book confronts the continually evolving nature of biomedical science education by providing a robust account of learning pedagogies and best practice for scholars and researchers in the field.

Rather than considering subdisciplines of biomedical science education separately, the volume takes a holistic approach and considers the complexities of teaching biomedical science as a whole, providing a nuanced overview of how a particular practice fits in such a course overall, as well as providing support for development within the reader's own subdiscipline. Ultimately, this holistic approach allows for expansive discussion of relevant pedagogical approaches that will directly inform innovations in the contemporary teaching of biomedical science education.

Novel in approach and underpinned by the latest in research innovations, this book will appeal to scholars, researchers and postgraduate students in the fields of medical education, higher education, and curriculum studies. Policy makers involved with health education and promotion as well as educational research will also benefit from the volume.

Donna Johnson is Course Director, Postgraduate Biomedical Science, Leeds Beckett University, UK.

Contemporary Pedagogies of Medical and Health Professions' Education

Series editors: Paul Crampton and John Tredinnick-Rowe

This novel series will focus on innovation and best practice in relation to curriculum design and teaching methodologies within the environments of medical schools, ultimately aiming to promote innovation in medical education. Books in the series offer cutting-edge examples of pedagogical techniques and practises through case studies and rigorous scholarship, and reflect subjects that medical schools are adapting in order to drive innovation such as the increasing role of patient-centred medicine or the expanding use of technology in medical curricula.

Themes identified in the series have international relevance given the similarities around educating medical students and their interaction with other clinical professions, and showcase novel research methodologies and frameworks to aid teaching and learning and preparedness of the next generation of clinical professionals.

Books in the series include:

Pedagogies of Biomedical Science
A Holistic Approach to Integrating Pedagogy Across the Curriculum
Edited by Donna Johnson

For more information about the series, please visit: www.routledge.com/Contemporary-Pedagogies-of-Medical-and-Health-Professions-Education/book-series/CPMHPE

Pedagogies of Biomedical Science

A Holistic Approach to Integrating Pedagogy Across the Curriculum

Edited by Donna Johnson

Routledge
Taylor & Francis Group

LONDON AND NEW YORK

First published 2024
by Routledge
4 Park Square, Milton Park, Abingdon, Oxon OX14 4RN

and by Routledge
605 Third Avenue, New York, NY 10158

Routledge is an imprint of the Taylor & Francis Group, an informa business

British Library Cataloguing-in-Publication Data
A catalogue record for this book is available from the British Library

ISBN: 978-1-032-46608-8 (hbk)
ISBN: 978-1-032-46964-5 (pbk)
ISBN: 978-1-003-38399-4 (ebk)

DOI: 10.4324/9781003383994

Typeset in Galliard
by SPi Technologies India Pvt Ltd (Straive)

Contents

**Innovative pedagogical approaches in biomedical
science education**   87

  6 Designing authentic learning practices for
     mid-degree biomedical science students   89
     KATHRYN DUDLEY AND TARA SABIR

  7 Effective student-centred assessment and feedback
     methods in biomedical science   106
     JESS HAIGH AND DONNA JOHNSON

  8 The capstone experience: creating changemakers   121
     DAVID I LEWIS

PART IV
Skills development and professional practice   **141**

  9 Developing key skills in science communication   143
     DONNA JOHNSON

 10 The value of Scicomm from the students' perspective –
     Building identity and professional values   156
     SARA SMITH AND MARTIN P KHECHARA

 11 Professional and career management: Developing
     employability and career skills for undergraduate
     and postgraduate biomedical science students   173
     GEORGINA LARKIN AND LIZ O'GARA

     Afterword   193

     Index   *195*

Contributors

Helen Battersby, NHS, UK

Helen Battersby is a Clinical Scientist in Genomics and has worked as a lecturer for Leeds Beckett University's Biomedical Science department. Helen believes that embedding healthcare scientists in academic positions not only supplies the students with real-world, relevant knowledge but also provides a unique insight for students to gain experience of professional standards. She has developed her career with active roles in training and leadership, working with regional Genomics centres in large teaching hospital NHS trusts. Helen has created a broad depth of experience in education and training within several NHS departments for an array of healthcare professionals at all levels and has worked on curriculum design for the National School of Healthcare Science Scientist Training Programme and Leeds Beckett University Biomedical Science courses. Helen is a fellow of the Higher Education Academy.

Avninder Bhambra, De Montfort University, UK

Dr Bhambra is currently an Associate Professor within the Faculty of Health and Life Sciences (HLS) at De Montfort University (DMU). Throughout his time at DMU, Dr Bhambra has taught across multiple HLS undergraduate and postgraduate degree programmes using an engaging and adaptive teaching and learning philosophy. He is an experienced Programme Leader where he successfully led the Institute of Biomedical Science (IBMS)-accredited BSc Biomedical Science programme. As an experienced academic with an interest in quality assurance, Dr Bhambra is actively involved in quality-related events with higher education institutes and accrediting bodies across the health and life science disciplines.

Kathryn Dudley, University of Wolverhampton, UK

Kathryn is a Health and Care Professions Council (HCPC)-registered Biomedical Scientist who worked for several years in the NHS as a Senior Biomedical Scientist and training officer before moving into academia. Kathryn now works as a Senior Lecturer in Biomedical Science at the University of Wolverhampton with additional responsibility for running NHS laboratory placements via the Applied Biomedical Science programme. Kathryn's research is pedagogically focused, having completed her doctoral thesis on stakeholder perceptions of the importance of patient outcomes within the Biomedical Scientist role. Kathryn is actively involved with the Institute of Biomedical Science (IBMS) as a registration portfolio verifier and is currently Chair of the IBMS Birmingham branch.

Jess Haigh, Leeds Beckett University, UK

Dr Jess Haigh is a Senior Lecturer in Biomedical Science at Leeds Beckett University. Jess studied for an undergraduate degree in Medical Sciences and a PhD in Neuroscience, both at the University of Leeds. She undertook postdoctoral positions at the University of California, Davis and the University of Leeds, using genomics techniques to probe neurodevelopmental disorders and metabolic disorders. Her research explores how insulin resistance develops following the consumption of a high-fat diet using cell culture models with the aim to identify novel therapeutic targets to counteract obesity and type 2 diabetes.

Jess delivers research-led teaching across BSc and MSc Biomedical Science modules with a focus on Pathology. She has an interest in improving authentic assessment practices for Biomedical Science to give students the opportunity to develop and showcase relevant skills for future jobs.

Ian Hurley, Leeds Beckett University, UK

Ian is a Senior Lecturer in the School of Health at Leeds Beckett University, teaching on the Undergraduate Biomedical Sciences courses, and is the Level 4 Lead. He teaches across a range of subjects, primarily genetics, biotechnology and research methods, and leads the Practical and Study Skills module which Level 4 students take in their first Semester. Ian also teaches in the Biomedical Sciences Masters programmes.

Having gained his PhD from the University of Liverpool, Ian worked as a researcher and lecturer in Biomedical Sciences at the University of Chester before moving to Leeds in September 2008.

Ian's research interests build on a background in applications of immunochemistry and molecular biology and current research focuses on the development of biomolecular speciation assays.

Ian's research is centred on the development of biomolecular speciation assays for the sensitive and selective detection of the species of origin of organic samples. Speciation assays can be developed for a number of applications. These assays involve the development of immunological and DNA-based methods for the detection of specific protein or DNA sequences within a sample.

Applications of these methods include the detection of fraudulent adulteration in food and drink, the identification of pathogenic bacteria and the forensic detection of blood traces at crime scenes and verification that the blood is human in origin.

Donna Johnson, Leeds Beckett University, UK

Donna is the Course Director for the Taught Postgraduate courses in Biomedical Science at Leeds Beckett University. Within this role she has led on IBMS and RSB accreditation for the masters courses. She has extensive experience teaching genetics and statistics at undergraduate and postgraduate levels. Her current interest is student support, in particular supporting the transition to masters level study. More recently, she has been investigating staff opinions on the impact of artificial intelligence in education and how AI can be integrated as a tool for student learning. She is a senior fellow of the HEA and a Chartered Science Teacher.

Martin P Khechara, University of Wolverhampton, UK

Martin Khechara is an Associate Professor for Engagement in science, technology, engineering and maths (STEM) at the University of Wolverhampton. Martin is a medical microbiologist, researcher and educator who has an international profile for his work in pedagogy for higher education. He is also a public engagement practitioner, science communicator, presenter, writer, director and science theatre performer who believes that study at university can change lives. Martin leads on the development of strategy for better outreach and public engagement for STEM subject areas for the University of Wolverhampton and is a champion of social change and actively works in the community as manager and creative director of the award-winning STEM Response Team. Through this group Martin has successfully managed a wide variety of high-value funded projects for outreach and public engagement and has used these to bring the magic of STEM subjects to those who need it the most.

Georgina Larkin, Leeds Beckett University, UK

Georgina Larkin is a Graduate Progression Consultant based in Leeds, West Yorkshire.

Following a first career as a communications consultant and subsequently freelance writer, editor and proofreader, Georgina joined the University of Leeds careers service in 2007 as a module administrator and qualified as a career adviser in 2014. In November 2014, Georgina joined Leeds Beckett University as a Careers Consultant, working predominantly with students from health and social sciences courses, including BSc and MSc Biomedical Science. From 2014 to 2022, Georgina worked closely with the BMS academic team to contribute to and deliver on the year-two Professional & Scientific Practice module.

Since January 2022, Georgina has worked as a Graduate Progression Consultant, working with final-year students and recent graduates, supporting them to transition from university to find fulfilling careers.

Georgina's specialist focus is on supporting students and graduates to identify and articulate their knowledge, skills and experience to empower them to move into jobs and careers that inspire them. She is a member of AGCAS

(Association of Graduate Careers Advisory Services) and delivered a workshop at the AGCAS conference in 2017. She is a Fellow of the Higher Education Academy.

David I Lewis, University of Leeds, UK

David (Dave) Lewis is a Senior Lecturer (Associate Professor) in Pharmacology and Bioethics at the University of Leeds, UK. He creates innovative, inspirational educational interventions that promote learner personal and professional development: capstone experiences; trans-national education for sustainable development opportunities; community-engaged experiential learning; professional education in research animal sciences and ethics. His main SOTL and pedagogical research interests are capstone projects, education for sustainable development and research animal sciences, animal welfare and ethics. He led the implementation of capstone projects across the UK Biosciences and increasing internationally, supporting educators across the world to introduce them into their undergraduate and Taught Postgraduate programmes. A Leeds Institute of Teaching Excellence Fellow, he is the University of Leeds' Curriculum Redefined Academic Lead for capstones, supporting their implementation into programmes across the University. Dave splits his time between the UK, EU, India and Africa. He is a Visiting Professor of Education for Professional Development or External Lecturer at Institutions in the UK, EU and Africa. He has received multiple prestigious awards for his educational activities from Advance HE, UK Physiological Society, British Pharmacological Society and UK Biochemical Society.

Alex Liversidge, Leeds Beckett University, UK

Alex has 20 years of post-graduate experience as a Biomedical Scientist within the private sector and NHS. Her specialist areas of Biomedical Science are Haematology and Blood Transfusion. Alex has previously been the Training Manager of the Blood Transfusion department at Leeds Teaching NHS Trust and Blood Bank Manager at Bradford Royal Infirmary. She joined as a lecturer in Blood Science within the Biomedical Science faculty at Leeds Beckett University in 2018.

Alex has previously researched the role of the Immature Reticulocyte Fraction (IRF) parameter of the Haematology analysers used in the NHS Pathology departments and has a current interest in Blood Transfusion.

Ismini Nakouti, Liverpool John Moores University, UK

Ismini was awarded a B.Sc. degree in Microbiology from the University of Liverpool in 2001. She went on to study for an M.Sc. degree in Industrial Biotechnology in 2002, and then a PhD in Applied Microbiology in 2008, both from Liverpool John Moores University (LJMU). She is a Microbiologist with eight years post-doctoral experience researching microbial interactions, biofilms and their natural products. She also has a Postgraduate Certificate in Learning and Teaching in Higher Education (2015, LJMU) and she is a Fellow of the Higher Education Academy.

Since 2015 she has been a Lecturer in Clinical Microbiology at the School of Pharmacy and Biomolecular Sciences, LJMU, developing an interest in medical diagnostics and applying her background to problems relevant to Civil Engineering and the Built Environment. She is the Section Lead for Microbial Natural Products in The Centre of Natural Products Discovery, LJMU, and an Editor for the Journal of Natural Products Discovery.

Ismini has been invited to disseminate her research at both national and international scientific meetings and she is regularly engaging in outreach activities giving talks and delivering workshops to schools and the local community. At LJMU she is a key team member of the Biomedical Science group and delivers a number of lectures in both Pharmacy and Biomolecular Sciences at undergraduate and postgraduate level.

Liz O'Gara, University of Wolverhampton, UK

Dr Elizabeth Ann O'Gara is a Principal Lecturer in the Faculty of Science and Engineering at the University of Wolverhampton. She has actively contributed to the provision of the Biomedical Science and Human Biology awards and has over 20 years of experience in teaching Medical Microbiology, Nutrition, and core and professional skills, in theoretical, practical and research modules. She has also taken on several leadership roles during her academic career including Faculty wide lead in employability and quality.

During her academic career she has specialised in the embedding of employability skills within awards, devising and delivering strategy in employability at the faculty level and has a strong background in curriculum review and design. She also has many years of experience working with the Institute of Biomedical Science and National School of Healthcare Science for accreditation of academic provisions.

She believes that teaching should be inclusive and that the curriculum should be designed to incorporate different learning styles, include authentic learning, and global examples, and that all programmes should prepare students to succeed.

Wayne Roberts, Leeds Beckett University, UK

Dr Wayne Roberts joined Leeds Beckett University in 2018 as the Course Director for Biomedical Science degree programmes. His research expertise is in the role platelets and platelet microparticles play in disease states.

Wayne graduated with a BSc (Hons) in Biomedical Sciences from the University of Bradford in 2004 before completing a PhD funded by Heart Research UK looking at the regulation of blood platelet activation. He next moved to Hull York Medical School for a British Heart Foundation-funded post-doctoral position, which focused on the regulation of platelet activation in health and disease. Following completion of a PGCE, he was employed as a lecturer in Medical Sciences at Bradford University. Wayne supervises a number of research projects at Leeds Beckett University examining how dysregulation of blood platelets can enhance disease progression.

Tara Sabir, Leeds Beckett University, UK

Dr Tara Sabir is a Senior Lecturer teaching Biochemistry in the Biomedical Sciences BSc course in the Faculty of Health & Social Sciences. She has a background in biochemistry and biophysics specifically in the field of single molecule fluorescence nanotechnology.

Following on from her PhD Tara spent a number of years working for small commercial spin-off companies offering DNA/RNA and protein characterisation services to industry before returning to academia as a postdoctoral research associate at the Photon Science Institute, University of Manchester. During her postdoctoral research she used multiparameter fluorescence detection (MFD) microscopy at the single molecule level to investigate the 3D global structure of 4-stranded fork structures (4-SF) of *E.coli.*

Tara continues to work in the field of single-molecule photonics and currently works on collaborative research projects with the University of Leeds Single Molecules Facility and the University of South Bohemia in České Budějovice.

Sara Smith, NHS Highland, UK

Sara Smith works for NHS Highland as the Lead for Developing Careers within Learning and Development. She originally trained as a biomedical scientist specialising in cellular pathology. Sara managed a busy pathology laboratory before moving into training and development and ran a Regional Cytology Training centre. After 16 years in the NHS she moved into Higher Education where she was course lead on both undergraduate and postgraduate courses in biomedical science and, prior to moving up to NHS Highland, course director for a Foundation Year to Medicine award. Sara's research focuses upon practitioner capability, addressing how we can support learning in and for the workplace.

Series editor foreword

Our intention with this book series is to explore fresh approaches, highlight points of difference and examine situations in which academics and researchers have sought to innovate to tackle problems and develop more effective sustainable solutions to teaching future healthcare workers.

More specifically, we have taken this fresh approach partly in reference to the many clinical professions experiencing crises in recruitment. Central government responses to this have involved increasing school places or placing great emphasis on increasing staff health and wellbeing during core and foundation training. *Contemporary Pedagogies of Medicine and Health* focuses on innovation and good practice in relation to curriculum design and teaching. Books in the series are segmented into two core types.

1 Pedagogies of individual subjects taught as part of a curriculum

   • E.g. Pedagogies for Biomedical Science

2 Pedagogies of topics or themes within clinical curriculums

   • E.g. Pedagogies of Widening Participation

In addition to texts on individual curriculum areas, the series will include books on themes that might emerge in several areas across a curriculum—for example, introducing social justice concerns, ethics or gender-related issues in medicine. A common feature of both formats is the variety of voices in chapters that create balanced monographs, which do not shy away from presenting differing stakeholder opinions or subjects that cross disciplinary boundaries. The series creates a space for critique and voicing of multiple points of view, which we believe are fundamental to drive forward meaningful progress in curriculum development. To this end, we welcome works co-authored with patients, students, and voices not typically heard in academic fields such as health and system regulators.

The international relevance of the series is driven by the fact that many workforce problems in medical and healthcare education are consistent across global borders such as increasing recruitment, retention of staff, sustainable delivery, technological advancement, preservation of wellbeing and many more. As a result, the series content is highly internationally relevant because it focuses on concerns that transcend national boundaries. Similarly, innovations and new approaches are required in all locations to continue to deliver high-quality education.

Consequently, the need to develop pedagogy within healthcare education to facilitate changes in teaching clinical subjects is a pressing current concern. The Lancet Commission, in their report on medical education, opined that medical school curricula were currently not fit to meet societal demands and were "*outdated and static*". This series offers a space for clinical tutors and academics to showcase how medical schools (and so curricula) can be made fit for the 21st century through the dissemination of evidence-based pedagogies for instruction, for which there is clearly a demand in terms of societal pressure but also a regulatory requirement.

The series' scope is broad and encourages submissions from underserved clinical subjects in terms of research and scholarship on education and pedagogy. We envisage cross-cutting themes in healthcare education and medical subjects but look to offer opportunities for specialisms that receive less limelight to showcase innovations, projects in allied healthcare and other clinical professions are very welcome. Moreover, there is scope for books to focus on new teaching methodologies present across different areas of medicine and other clinical subjects combined.

We believe this series will interest anyone involved in the development of healthcare professions because of the salience (and need) of education, workforce, and regulatory developments as we all attempt to increase the quantity and quality of trainees entering a health service.

The first book in the series is Donna Johnson's pioneering work, which brings to life the pedagogical techniques used in the delivery of biomedical science education. Medical education literature often overlooks this foundational subject pertinent to all clinical courses. Consequently, we are glad to present a source material for educators and tutors that fills a core gap in provision.

The publication is true to the series' goals of being both practical and innovative. It makes extensive use of case studies, allowing the reader to follow their development whilst showcasing contemporary approaches to teaching biomedical science. The chapters flow naturally, starting with curriculum development and move towards a focus on careers in the later part of the book. Hence, Donna Johnson and her co-authors have produced valuable insights that are useful for innovative delivery but also consider the longer-term picture of where graduates will go. We see this book as being a staple of the literature on biomedical science education for many years to come and hope you enjoy reading it as much as we did.

Introduction

At the heart of biomedical science education is the need to impart a comprehensive understanding of the human body, exploring its functions in states of health and disease. This educational journey is not a superficial overview but a deep dive into the complex biological systems that define human life. Curricula encompass a range of foundational subjects, each playing a pivotal role in shaping a student's understanding of the workings of the body. This involves delving into subjects such as biochemistry, cell biology, genetics, immunology, microbiology, and pathology among others. These foundational subjects are crucial for students to understand the complex interactions and processes that occur within the body and through these subjects, biomedical science education provides students with a holistic understanding of the human body. The knowledge gained from these foundational subjects is not isolated; rather, it is interlinked, reflecting the interconnected nature of biological systems. This integrated approach is vital, ultimately preparing students for careers in biomedical research, healthcare, and beyond.

A distinguishing feature of biomedical science education is the balanced emphasis it places on both theoretical knowledge and practical skills. This dual focus is fundamental, as students need to not only understand theoretical concepts but also how to apply them in practical contexts. Practical sessions are therefore integral to the curriculum, serving as essential platforms where students can apply their theoretical learning in real-world scenarios and learn how to design experiments, handle sophisticated equipment, and conduct various procedures that are crucial in biomedical research.

This practical approach is not just about learning techniques; it's about developing a mindset and skill set that are essential in the biomedical field. Problem-solving is one such skill. In the laboratory, students often encounter unexpected results or technical challenges. Addressing these situations requires them to think critically, hypothesise possible reasons, and find solutions. Analytical thinking is another critical skill developed through practical sessions. Students learn to analyse and interpret data which is a crucial skill for making sense of experimental results and translating them into meaningful conclusions. In the context of biomedical science, where data interpretation can have

DOI: 10.4324/9781003383994-1

significant implications for research and patient care, the ability to analyse and interpret data accurately and critically is vital.

As well as foundational skills and knowledge, curricula also introduce students to the research process encompassing various critical stages from hypothesis formation to the interpretation of results.

Hypothesis formation is often the starting point in the research process. This involves identifying a research question and formulating a hypothesis based on existing scientific knowledge. The curriculum teaches students how to craft a well-grounded hypothesis, which requires critical thinking and a deep understanding of the subject matter. Experimental design is another key component. The curriculum focuses on teaching students how to design experiments that are methodologically sound and capable of effectively testing their hypotheses. This includes understanding how to control variables, determine sample sizes, and select appropriate methods and techniques. A well-designed experiment is essential for obtaining reliable and interpretable results, and students learn to anticipate potential challenges and confounding factors in their experimental design. Data analysis and interpretation are important steps in the research process too, where students learn to apply statistical methods to analyse and interpret their data. This involves not just the application of statistical techniques but also the ability to discern which methods are most appropriate for different types of data and research questions. Students also learn how to interpret their findings in the context of the broader scientific literature, understanding how their results contribute to the existing body of knowledge.

Biomedical science education is intricately linked with the healthcare sector, reflecting its practical applications and real-world relevance. The curriculum is designed not just to impart scientific knowledge but also to align closely with the needs and expectations of the healthcare industry. This alignment is essential in preparing students for a range of roles that directly impact health and wellbeing. It also responds to changes in healthcare needs and practices. The healthcare sector is constantly evolving, influenced by factors such as emerging health challenges, shifts in disease patterns, and advancements in medical treatments and diagnostics and biomedical science education adapts to these changes by updating its content to reflect the current landscape of healthcare. This dynamic approach to education ensures that students are not only well-versed in the foundational principles of biomedical science but also adept at applying this knowledge in a rapidly changing world. They learn to be adaptable, a trait that is increasingly valuable in a professional environment where change is the only constant. The evolving nature of the curriculum fosters a mindset of lifelong learning among students as well. They come to understand that education does not end with graduation; rather, it is a continuous process of updating and expanding their knowledge and skills.

This book's creation is deeply rooted in acknowledging the complex nature of biomedical science education. Biomedical science stands out for its complexity and dynamism, a reflection of the ever-evolving scientific landscape and the diverse challenges it presents. This complexity is not just academic; it extends to the practical realms that students will navigate post-graduation. Consequently, the design of a biomedical science curriculum demands more than academic rigour; it requires a curriculum that resonates with real-world scenarios, equipping graduates with the skills and knowledge to thrive in professional settings. We consider several key themes that support educators in producing an excellent biomedical science curriculum:

- Curriculum design rationale and principles: The curriculum serves as a key academic document that defines the structure, content, rationale, and vision of a biomedical science course. It must cater to the needs of the profession and prepare students for diverse career paths in biomedical science and related fields. It should be fit for purpose, assuring stakeholders of its quality and relevance in higher education. Courses should align with intended learning objectives, ensuring that assessments and teaching activities are designed to achieve specific, measurable goals. Feedback on assessments is crucial for student development.
- Content and skills development: Biomedical science education must provide a strong foundation in basic sciences and the fundamental disciplines of biomedical science, both in health and disease. It should include lab skills training, research skills training, and foster employability through professional development, transferable skills, and communication skills.
- Inclusivity and diversity: Recognising the increasingly diverse student cohorts, biomedical science education should accommodate and appreciate these differences, allowing all students to achieve their best. This includes using alternative learning formats, promoting collaboration among diverse student populations, and creating a respectful and inclusive learning environment.
- Authenticity and adaptability: Biomedical science education must remain relevant and incorporate experiential learning opportunities. Teaching methods like case studies bridge theory with practice, and hands-on research and interdisciplinary collaboration are emphasised. Regular updates to the curriculum are necessary to keep pace with advancements in biomedical technology and changes within pathology units in the NHS.
- Professional standards and employability: Adherence to professional body benchmarks and standards, such as those set by the IBMS, the RSB, and the QAA, is critical. This ensures that students are prepared for professional certifications and have enhanced employability.

In essence, this book seeks to offer a blueprint for designing and delivering a curriculum that is academically rigorous, professionally relevant, and attuned to the development of critical skills needed for success in the biomedical field. Through this approach, the book aims to contribute to the evolution of biomedical science education, shaping a generation of graduates who are not only knowledgeable but also adept at navigating the challenges of the biomedical landscape.

Part I

Foundations of biomedical science education

1   Curriculum design

Avninder Bhambra and Donna Johnson

What do we need from a biomedical science degree?

There are two key groups of students for a biomedical science degree, those wishing to pursue a career in the NHS as a Biomedical Scientist and those with a more general interest, we need to provide a meaningful suite of degrees to meet the needs of both these groups of students. The importance of curriculum design in biomedical science education lies in its ability to prepare students for successful careers in biomedical science and related fields. When our curricula are well-designed, they allow our students to acquire the necessary knowledge and competencies to excel in their chosen careers and adapt to the ever-evolving biomedical landscape[1].

One of the critical aspects of curriculum design is ensuring relevance and authenticity. By providing content that is timely and relevant, students will develop a deep understanding of the topics covered and will be better equipped with practical skills that are valued in the workforce. We should also incorporate research and experiential learning opportunities to help students connect theoretical knowledge with practical applications[2,3]. Another important factor is helping students to develop their critical thinking and problem-solving skills. By including active learning activities, such as case studies, projects, and inquiry-based learning, students are encouraged to think critically, being able to analyse complex problems and develop innovative solutions[4].

Interdisciplinarity is crucial in biomedical science. Biomedical Scientists will often need to collaborate with colleagues from various fields, so to better prepare students for this we need to expose our students to different perspectives and encourage collaborative projects. When we do this, they learn how to effectively communicate and work with professionals from a range of other disciplines.

We use our curriculum design processes in order to ensure we meet professional body benchmarks and standards. This is vital if we are to ensure that our students are adequately prepared for professional certifications, which can enhance their employability. It also helps to establish a strong foundation in ethics and professionalism, which are vital for a successful career in biomedical science[5,6].

DOI: 10.4324/9781003383994-3

Considerations for curriculum design

When designing curricula for biomedical science there are several key principles: assessment and feedback, relevance and authenticity, supporting interdisciplinary learning, and inclusivity and diversity[7].

Aligning assessments and teaching activities with intended learning objectives ensures that the curriculum is designed to achieve specific objectives, which are clearly defined and measurable. Here we need to identify the knowledge and skills that we want our students to acquire by the end of their course then tailor the content, activities, and assessments to meet these goals[8]. The way we approach providing feedback to assessments is also important. Feedback is traditionally scored relatively low in student satisfaction surveys and the prevailing opinion is that this is at least in part due to differences between staff and student perceptions of what feedback is and how it should be used. If we are clear in our discussion of this and where possible provide formative opportunities then we can support our students' development off the back of their feedback.

Ensuring relevance and authenticity in the biomedical science curriculum is vital for preparing students to transition seamlessly from university to the workplace. By designing curriculum content that reflects relevant real-world applications within biomedical science, we can equip our students with the knowledge and skills they need in order to excel in their careers. Case studies are a good example of a teaching tool that allows students to apply theoretical concepts to real-life situations. They can help students develop a better understanding of the complexities and ethical considerations involved in research and clinical practice. This approach also encourages the development of critical thinking skills, as students must evaluate the evidence, identify relevant factors, and justify their conclusions[9,10]. Using case studies and similar approaches in teaching can also help to support interdisciplinary learning. We can include information from a range of sources that students then need to interpret and integrate into their answers[11].

We have increasingly diverse cohorts[12]; students come to university at undergraduate and postgraduate levels with a range of abilities and educational, social, and cultural backgrounds and we need to design courses that appreciate these differences and allow all our students to achieve their best. Integrating consideration of inclusivity and diversity should be integral to our curriculum design processes as it not only enhances the educational experiences of all students but also promotes a sense of belonging and engagement. By including content that reflects the contributions and experiences of individuals from various cultural, ethnic, and gender backgrounds, students can also appreciate the value of diverse perspectives[13].

If we adapt our teaching methods to accommodate different learning styles and preferences, we can help to ensure that all students can effectively engage with our materials. Alternative formats, such as captioned videos, audio recordings, or translated texts, as well as support services, like tutoring or assessment accommodations, can facilitate this inclusivity. Designing activities and assignments that encourage collaboration and interaction among students from diverse backgrounds promotes learning from one another, the development of cross-cultural communication skills, and a sense of belonging within the classroom[14].

Creating a supportive learning environment is essential for student success, especially in the context of increasingly diverse student populations, this helps all students feel valued and engaged in their learning. We need to set and model clear behavioural expectations to help students understand the importance of treating one another with respect and dignity. Addressing microaggressions is another important aspect of creating an inclusive learning environment. Microaggressions are subtle, often unintentional actions or comments that convey bias or prejudice towards marginalised groups[15]. We need to be proactive in identifying and addressing these, both by raising awareness about their impact and by providing guidance on how to avoid or respond to them in a constructive manner. It is also important to encourage an open dialogue about diversity and inclusivity because this can help to create a learning environment where students feel comfortable discussing their experiences and concerns[16,17].

When considering specific content within the curriculum for a biomedical science degree there are three core elements we should consider:

1 Knowledge

- A strong foundation in basic sciences
- A strong foundation in the fundamental disciplines of biomedical science in health and disease

2 Skills

- Lab skills training
- Research skills training

3 Employability

- Professional development
- Transferrable skills
- Communication skills

Knowledge

Students will come into a biomedical science degree with at least some science experience, but this will be varied across the cohort in terms of type of qualification and content. This diversity necessitates a comprehensive first-year curriculum to bring all students to a common foundation of understanding, preparing them for the more advanced concepts they will cover at levels five and six.

Integrating basic sciences such as maths, biology, physics, and chemistry into early modules can be beneficial, as these disciplines form the foundation for a successful biomedical science education. By providing clear connections to the relevance of these subjects and their future applications, students can better understand the importance of a strong foundation in basic sciences.

Biomedical science offers multiple opportunities to teach basic sciences through real-world examples. For instance, physics can be taught in the context of imaging techniques such as MRI and X-ray, chemistry can be explored through lab tests and diagnostics, and maths can be integrated into the analysis of biomedical data. Biology is inherently embedded in most biomedical science modules, providing a seamless connection to the subject matter.

Developing knowledge and understanding of fundamental biomedical science disciplines can be achieved through subject-specific modules that build upon one another throughout the degree program. One potential approach is to introduce core concepts at level four, explore their applications in health at level five, and delve more deeply into clinical applications and disease contexts at level six. This progressive structure ensures that students have a clear understanding of the knowledge development across the degree path and can make connections between previous and future modules (Table 1.1).

Skills

It is essential to develop lab and research skills throughout a biomedical science degree and we can take a similarly progressive approach as we do for developing knowledge. By doing so, students are better equipped to handle the increasing complexity of lab techniques. It also ensures that students are well-prepared for a career in biomedical science, where practical skills and hands-on experience are essential for success.

At level four, students will be introduced to the basic lab skills and methods essential for biomedical science. The focus here is on familiarising students with the lab environment, equipment, safety requirements, and standard operating procedures. At level five, students will further develop their lab skills by learning and applying more advanced techniques specific to biomedical science. They should begin to integrate and apply their theoretical knowledge to perform experiments and analyse their results. Skills refinement is the goal at level six. We want students to be engaging in complex and specialised experiments and they generally do so in the context of their research projects. Students are expected to design, execute, and interpret experiments while demonstrating critical thinking and problem-solving skills.

In terms of research skills, at level four, students will be introduced to the fundamental concepts of research and the scientific method. This is combined with developing their skills in reading scientific literature and interpreting data. At level five, students should be beginning to integrate their theoretical knowledge and basic research skills in the context of experimental design and more thoroughly be able to consider the ethical implications of research. Level six is again about refinement and increasingly independent application of skills as a component of their research projects.

Table 1.1 Progressive education in biomedical science sub-discipline

Level	Disciplines and example topics						
	Anatomy and physiology	Microbiology	Immunology	Biochemistry	Genetics and molecular biology	Cell biology	Pharmacology
4	Basic human anatomy, organ systems, and physiological functions	Introduction to microorganisms, their classification, and basic structure	Overview of the immune system, innate and adaptive immunity	Basic principles of biochemistry, biomolecules, and metabolic pathways	Fundamentals of genetics, DNA structure, replication, and gene expression	Basic cell structure, function, and cellular processes	Introduction to pharmacology, drug classification, and mechanisms of action
5	Homeostasis, physiological adaptations, and common disorders	Microbial growth, metabolism, and mechanisms of pathogenicity	Molecular and cellular mechanisms of immune response and regulation	Enzyme function, regulation, and biochemical signalling pathways	Principles of inheritance, genetic mutations, and molecular techniques	Cell signalling, cell cycle, and mechanisms of cell differentiation and specialisation	Pharmacokinetics, pharmacodynamics, and drug-receptor interactions
6	Advanced topics in human physiology, pathological conditions, and clinical interventions	Diagnostic microbiology, antimicrobial therapies, and emerging infectious	Immunopathology, immunodeficiencies, and clinical applications of immunotherapy	Advanced topics in metabolism, bioenergetics, and the role of biochemistry in disease	Genomics, epigenetics, and applications in genetic diagnostics and therapies	Advanced topics in cellular pathology, cancer biology, and stem cell research	Advanced topics in drug development, personalised medicine, and pharmacogenomics

Employability

Including career development in our curricula has a proven positive impact on student employability[18]. Preparing students for successful and satisfying careers in biomedical science involves a multifaceted approach that includes developing employability skills and relevant competencies, facilitating networking opportunities and providing career guidance and support. This is essential for ensuring that our students are well-equipped for their future careers. Development of transferrable skills should be well integrated into the curriculum and providing opportunities to gain hands-on experience through placements, or research projects can help them develop practical skills relevant to their field[19,20].

One thing that can be particularly difficult for students to do independently is to build their professional networks. Most biomedical science degrees contain professional development modules and these are good places to embed sessions to help our students with this. We can use activities such as conferences and professional seminars and invite guest lecturers and then facilitate opportunities for students to talk to the professionals in an informal setting[21].

Providing career guidance is another important aspect of preparing students for their careers. We should be working hand in hand with our central career services to signpost students to the resources available and to take advantage of the wealth of experience our career advisors have. Our career advisors possess valuable knowledge about the job market, and sharing this information with students can help them make informed decisions about their career paths and better prepare for the job market.

What about at masters level?

At masters level, the core elements of the curriculum need to be increased to reflect the advanced level of study and associated career aspirations of our students:

1 Knowledge

- A deep understanding of advanced biomedical science concepts
- Comprehensive knowledge of biomedical science in health and disease

2 Skills

- Advanced lab skills training
- Advanced research skills training

3 Employability

- Advanced professional development
- Enhanced transferrable skills
- Advanced communication skills

Knowledge

At masters level, students should already possess a comprehensive understanding of the basic sciences as well as a strong foundation in the fundamental disciplines of biomedical science. Their previous qualifications will differ, so there will be a need for a curriculum that acknowledges this diversity while pushing students to greater depths of understanding. Depending on the specific focus of the course, students will be delving into more advanced aspects of the concepts, for example moving from genetics to genomics and its application across a range of disciplines. Despite the more focused nature of masters course, it is still important to integrate knowledge from multiple areas so students can better understand the more complex biomedical systems they will cover.

A vital aspect at masters level is the further development of critical analysis skills and how these are applied. The ability to critically evaluate scientific literature forms the cornerstone of postgraduate education. At this level, students are expected to dissect journal articles in order to assess the quality of the research methods, the validity of data, the soundness of the analysis, and the relevance of conclusions drawn. Not only does this process facilitate comprehension of cutting-edge developments, it also sharpens students' understanding of effective research design and methodology which they can then apply in their research projects.

While masters courses tend to be a year-long, the progressive structure is still relevant, but should be adjusted to fit the course length and content. Students will come to the course with a solid grasp of fundamental biomedical science disciplines and to support this, at the beginning of the course, we can introduce them to more specialised areas of study such as molecular biology, genomics, proteomics, bioinformatics, systems biology, etc though the exact specialties will depend on the focus of the course. At this level, students would explore the advanced theory, techniques, and current research within these areas. Moving to the next level, we can emphasise the practical applications of the specialised areas and broaden the focus to include an interdisciplinary understanding, exploring how different areas of biomedical science can be integrated to solve complex health issues. At the final level, we can delve even deeper into the clinical applications and disease contexts of the specialised areas. This could involve a detailed study of a range of aspects such as the pathophysiology of various diseases, the development of diagnostic methods, treatments, or preventative measures.

Skills

At masters level, the development of lab and research skills takes on a new level of complexity, focusing on advanced techniques and the integration of various aspects of biomedical science combined with greater independence. The aim is not only to equip students with the necessary technical skills but also to prepare them for the challenges they will encounter in their professional or academic careers.

For lab skills, the first level of a masters course should transition from general lab skills to more advanced, specialised techniques that are integral to the field of biomedical science. These can range from techniques in molecular biology and genetics to bioinformatics and next-generation sequencing, among others. The focus should not just be on mastering these techniques but on understanding their underlying principles and applications. The second level should build on these skills, integrating them into a broader scientific context. Students should be able to apply their advanced lab skills to complex, real-world problems, combining their technical abilities with their theoretical knowledge. Here, students should be expected to independently design and execute experiments, as well as interpret and analyse the resulting data. The final level should be characterised by a significant degree of independence and sophistication in lab skills. As part of their research projects, students should be conducting complex, specialised experiments, using a range of advanced techniques. They should also demonstrate a high level of critical thinking and problem-solving skills, as they design, execute, and interpret their own experiments.

In terms of research skills, masters level requires a significant degree of depth and sophistication. The first level should introduce students to advanced concepts in research, including experimental design, grant writing, and ethical considerations and this should be integrated with the development of their critical analysis skills. Following on from this, students should begin to integrate their theoretical knowledge with their research skills. This includes designing their own experiments, looking at how applications for grants are produced and the importance of research ethics and health and safety. If possible, it is also beneficial to provide opportunities for students to be given opportunities to participate in collaborative research projects, allowing them to experience and navigate the dynamics of team-based research which is likely to be something they will experience frequently in their careers. The final level should be characterised by a high level of independence in research. Students should be significantly involved in their own research projects where they should be responsible for all stages of the project as far as possible, this not only enhances their research skills but also prepares them more effectively for the workplace.

Employability

Incorporating career development at masters level often involves a more targeted approach than at the undergraduate level. It necessitates a stronger focus on the unique career aspirations of students, fostering advanced skills and competencies that align with their specific professional goals in biomedical science. Equally important is the cultivation of professional networking, research opportunities, and individualised career guidance. We need to ensure students develop advanced transferable skills such as leadership and project management or advanced data analysis and technical writing. These skills can be developed through problem-based learning, team projects, or research work, and should be fully integrated into the curriculum.

Gaining real-world experience or understanding is important to prepare masters students for work, while it can often be difficult to incorporate work experience within a masters course, if we can get involvement from those already working, we can at least provide students with additional perspectives and insights into the practical aspects of the biomedical science field. Indeed, integrating industry professionals into the masters curriculum can significantly enhance students' understanding of the real-world applications of their studies, and offer valuable networking opportunities. The involvement of industry professionals can take many forms. They could be invited as guest lecturers or workshop facilitators to discuss current trends or challenges in the field, providing students with firsthand insights into real-world aspects. These sessions can cover a wide range of topics and could present case studies from the workplace, demonstrating how theoretical concepts are applied in practical settings. If practicable, these professionals could also serve as mentors for students or their research projects, offering guidance and feedback throughout the process. This would provide students with an invaluable opportunity to gain a deeper understanding of the complexities and nuances of professional work in biomedical science, as well as to learn from the experiences and expertise of established professionals. Another effective strategy is the organisation of career fairs, where students can interact directly with representatives from various companies. This not only gives students an overview of potential career paths, but also helps them build connections that could lead to job opportunities. Activities like these tie in well with the development of professional networking skills, facilitating informal interactions between students and professionals can help them expand their network and gain insights into potential career paths.

Most masters courses have a professional development-focused module, and this is a good place to integrate the development of employability skills. We should consider getting our central careers services involved too, they have a range of specific skills that will be valuable for our students and will be able to signpost them to the wide range of career development resources an institution provides. Career advisors are well-versed in the latest job market trends, employment opportunities, and the specific requirements of various roles within the biomedical science field. They can provide invaluable advice to students about choosing suitable career paths and understanding the skills and qualifications sought by employers.

Integration of professional body benchmarks

Recent years have seen the popularity of biomedical science degrees increase, with rising student cohorts from both home and international settings. The Biomedical Science title is protected and can only be used by professionals registered with the Health and Care Professions Council (HCPC), so it must be clear to incoming students how they can achieve such standing. In order to become a Biomedical Scientist, candidates need to demonstrate evidence and the ability to meet the HCPC standards of proficiency. This is usually shown through a combination of academic and clinical training, where the former involves the completion of an Institute of Biomedical Science (IBMS) accredited degree which meets the HCPC standards of education and training, and the latter includes the completion of a Registration Training Portfolio (RTP) in an IBM approved laboratory. In most cases, the RTP is undertaken during a significant period of clinical training, and upon successful completion and verification, the IBMS Certificate of Competence is awarded. The abovementioned achievements demonstrate the holder to be fit for practice and eligible to apply for professional registration with HCPC.

IBMS-accredited degree programmes

As mentioned earlier in this chapter, the design of degree programmes is referenced through Subject Benchmark Statements (SBS) written by subject specialists and published through the Quality Assurance Agency for Higher Education (QAA)[22]. In March 2023, a revised biomedical science SBS was released which for the first time, differentiated between guidance for biomedical science and biomedical sciences degrees. However, if the eventual destination of students is HCPC registration as a Biomedical Scientist, degree programmes should be designed with reference to the biomedical science SBS, and importantly, accredited by the IBMS[23,24], an approved education provider by the HCPC.

Biomedical science is a complex discipline at the interface between biology and chemistry. There is an expectancy for graduates to be able to connect and integrate knowledge from a range of applicable topics, to demonstrate and expand understanding of the investigation, diagnosis and monitoring of human health and disease, as well as therapeutic strategies for patient treatment. Programmes should demonstrate a clear integration of clinical pathology with reference to human disorders, disease processes, their investigation and therapeutic contribution to patient care. In order to meet this, degree programmes should have clearly articulated methods for the delivery of clinical laboratory specialisms as set out in the Criteria and Requirements for the Accreditation of BSc (Hons) Degrees in Biomedical Science (Table 1.2). Specialisms have traditionally been recognised as cellular pathology, clinical biochemistry, clinical immunology, haematology, transfusion science, clinical genetics, and medical microbiology, however, reconfiguration within pathology units in the NHS has seen change to Blood Science, Cellular Science, Tissue Pathology, Infections and Molecular Science.

In addition to taught specialisms, a biomedical science degree must incorporate an independent research project which is typically undertaken at level 6 with a minimum of 20 credits. The research project should be a 'must pass' component where compensatory mechanisms of student progression do not apply. Projects can be laboratory or non-laboratory based, however, if the latter approach is undertaken there must be clear evidence of data generation, critical analyses, and application of results which can be through systematic reviews and bioinformatics type projects but not a literature review.

Table 1.2 Clinical specialisms – Criteria and requirements for the accreditation of BSc (Hons) Degrees in biomedical science

Cellular pathology	Clinical biochemistry	Clinical immunology	Haematology	Transfusion science	Clinical Genetics	Medical microbiology
The gross structure and ultrastructure of normal cells and tissues and the structural changes that may occur during disease	The range and methods used for the collection of clinical samples that may be subjected to biochemical analysis	The principles of the function and measurement of effectors of the immune response	The structure, function, and production of blood cells	The genetics, inheritance, structure and role of red cell antigens	Genomic, transcriptomic, and proteomic methods used to analyse and study human chromosomes and DNA	The pathogenic mechanisms of a range of organisms
Reproductive science including infertility and embryology	The principles and applications of biochemical investigations used for screening, diagnosis, treatment, and monitoring of disease, including near-patient testing	The causes and consequences of diseases associated with abnormal immune function, neoplastic diseases, and transplantation reactions together with their diagnosis, treatment, and monitoring	The regulation of normal haemostasis	Immune-mediated destruction of blood cells	The application of molecular biology and bioinformatics in medicine	Public health microbiology

(Continued)

Table 1.2 (Continued)

Cellular pathology	Clinical biochemistry	Clinical immunology	Haematology	Transfusion science	Clinical Genetics	Medical microbiology
The preparation of cells and tissues for microscopic examination	Therapeutic drug monitoring and investigation of substance abuse.	Principles and practice of immunological techniques used for screening, diagnosis, treatment, and monitoring of disease prophylaxis and immunotherapy.	Nature and diagnosis of anaemias, haematological malignancies, haemorrhagic, and thrombotic diseases	The preparation, storage, and use of blood components	Pharmacogenetics and personalised medicine	Principles and practice of techniques for screening, diagnosis, treatment and monitoring of a range of infectious diseases, including isolation and identification of microorganisms
The principles and applications of visualisation and imaging techniques, including microscopy, to aid diagnosis and treatment selection.			Principles and practice of haematological techniques used for screening, diagnosis, treatment, and monitoring of disease.	The selection of appropriate blood components for transfusion and possible adverse effects.	Principles and practice of techniques used for genetic testing for screening, diagnosis, treatment and monitoring of disease and associated ethical issues.	Prevention and control of infection, including anti-microbial and anti-viral therapy (including drug resistance).

Another critical aspect of programme design for an accredited biomedical science degree relates to management and resources to ensure the curriculum remains current with industry standards. It is common practice for programme teams to include visiting lecturers from Biomedical Scientists in practice, delivering on a range of activities from lectures to laboratory classes. Regular employer liaison committee meetings also provide a forum for supporting the development of programmes, which serves as a powerful tool in keeping content pertinent and current to the discipline.

Postgraduate provision

Currently, a number of UK HE organisations provide postgraduate biomedical science programmes, which typically involve the transition from undergraduate offerings of the same. Unlike the latter, a QAA SBS specifically for a masters level programme is not available, but guidance should still be taken from documents including the UK Quality Code for Higher Education, the QAA Biomedical Science SBS, and the IBMS Criteria and Requirements for the Accreditation of MSc Degrees in Biomedical Science.

With reference to the UK Quality Code for Higher Education, in summary masters degrees are awarded to students who have demonstrated and are able to show the following:

- a systematic understanding of knowledge, and a critical awareness of current problems informed by the forefront of their field/area of professional practice
- a comprehensive understanding of techniques applicable to their own research or advanced scholarship
- originality in the application of knowledge, a practical understanding of how techniques of research and enquiry are used to generate and interpret knowledge in the discipline, and the ability to critically evaluate current research and advanced scholarship in the discipline
- to evaluate and critique methodologies and where appropriate, to propose new hypotheses.

The QAA Biomedical Science SBS details benchmark standards which should be demonstrable by graduates completing a Biomedical Science/Sciences MSc programme. These standards largely reflect the ability of graduates to work independently and to combine/explore multiple methods of investigation to reach complex conclusions with further examples as follows:

- Interrogate and integrate diverse sources of scientific literature alongside other information sources, in order to design and develop methods for investigation and analysis, including in areas at the forefront of knowledge and outside their current specialist knowledge.
- Project planning, including, as appropriate, evaluation of ethics, hazards, environmental effects, sustainability, and appreciation of costs.

- Development of advanced experimental and investigative skills as appropriate for the project.
- Discussion of the background, context, methods, results, and potential impact of a significant research project.

The IBMS Criteria and Requirements for the Accreditation of MSc Degrees in biomedical science details further specific requirements of programmes that wish to embark on IBMS accreditation. MSc Programmes may encapsulate the broader biomedical science discipline or show a single focus related to the key specialist areas. It is noteworthy to say that programmes are not specifically accredited for graduates to use as a qualification suitable for registration with the HCPC so this should again be explicit to those wishing to embark on such programmes.

The curriculum should show students being exposed to a sound knowledge base which supports learning of current and future aspects of the discipline in the working environment e.g., areas associated with quality assurance and leadership and management. The curriculum structure should consider no more than 25% of undergraduate level content with the proposed MSc programme(s) and for students to complete a significant research project (typically laboratory-based) which constitutes at least one-third of the total credits being awarded for the MSc programme. The development and structure of the curriculum should also be informed by suitably experienced Biomedical Scientists to ensure that there is a contribution from the profession for the delivery of the key laboratory specialties, as well as employer liaison committees to evidence the academic-professional integration.

The design and delivery of a biomedical science course, whether undergraduate or postgraduate, is a nuanced and multifaceted endeavour that requires a keen understanding of the complexities of the discipline and a commitment to producing well-rounded, capable graduates. The curriculum must remain relevant, incorporate experiential learning opportunities, and foster the development of critical thinking and problem-solving abilities, all while maintaining rigorous professional standards. Authenticity and relevance are the mainstays of such curricula, as it's important to prepare students for the real-world challenges they will face in the workforce. This is achieved by carefully curating content, using teaching methods such as case studies that bridge theory and practice, and providing ample opportunities for hands-on research and interdisciplinary collaboration. Ensuring that the content, activities, and assessments are in line with specific, measurable learning objectives is also a key aspect of the curriculum design process.

Acknowledging and celebrating diversity within student cohorts is also central to effective curriculum design. By making inclusivity a cornerstone of the educational experience, we not only enrich the learning environment but also empower students from various backgrounds to flourish. This is realised through a combination of alternative formats for learning materials, collaboration and interaction among diverse student populations, and by creating a respectful and inclusive learning environment.

Adherence to professional body benchmarks and standards such as those set by the IBMS and the QAA is crucial. These bodies guide and shape the design of biomedical science courses, ensuring that students are fully prepared for professional certifications and enhancing their employability.

It is crucial too, to adapt to the evolving landscape of biomedical science, particularly considering advancements in biomedical technology and changes within pathology units in the NHS. By regularly reviewing and updating our programmes, we can ensure the curriculum remains pertinent and current to the discipline. In sum, the primary objective of a well-designed biomedical science curriculum should be to cultivate competent, ethical, and adaptable professionals capable of navigating the complex and rapidly changing biomedical science field. It is our role as educators to make this possible and shape the future of biomedical science education.

Case study: Equality, diversity, and inclusion in curriculum design

In the most recent version of the QAA Benchmarks for biomedical science[25] there were new themes for consideration:

- Equality, diversity, and inclusion (EDI).
- Accessibility and the needs of disabled students.
- Education for sustainable development.
- Employability, entrepreneurship, and enterprise education.

The principles of EDI carry considerable ethical and practical significance, particularly in the design of curricula. From an ethical standpoint, education serves as a powerful tool for social mobility and empowerment and so it is important that the educational framework is constructed to be accessible and beneficial to all, irrespective of their background, gender, ethnicity, or other distinguishing characteristics. Failing to integrate EDI into curriculum design could perpetuate social inequalities, as it might inadvertently favour one group over another in terms of the relevance and applicability of the course material. EDI is crucial for enriching the educational experience itself. A diverse and inclusive curriculum introduces students to a broad array of perspectives and ways of thinking. This not only stimulates intellectual curiosity but also encourages critical thinking, a skill highly valued in academic and professional settings. By learning to consider various viewpoints, students are better equipped to engage in nuanced debate and problem-solving.

On a more pragmatic note, we live in an increasingly globalised world where the ability to understand and interact with people from diverse backgrounds is not just an asset – it's a necessity. The workplace is becoming more diverse, and employers are increasingly seeking individuals who can navigate this complexity effectively. In this context, a curriculum that incorporates EDI principles helps prepare students for real-world challenges, enabling them to be more adaptable and effective in varied settings.

There is an increasing body of evidence to suggest that diverse classrooms and inclusive teaching strategies improve academic outcomes for all students, not just those from marginalised communities. For instance, studies have shown that students in diverse educational environments often demonstrate improved cognitive skills, including critical thinking and problem-solving. Therefore, prioritising EDI in curriculum design can be seen as a pathway to higher academic achievement and better long-term outcomes for students.

While aspects of EDI will already be embedded across all curricula, it may be that these factors have not been explicitly considered during the curriculum design process. Here we consider one approach to integrating EDI into the design of a final year module on Clinical Immunology.

When initially designing or revising the module, it's crucial to undertake a rigorous review of existing course materials. Textbooks, journal articles, and case studies should be scrutinised to ensure they represent a diverse array of voices and perspectives. For instance, if you find that the course predominantly relies on research conducted on male subjects or focuses solely on Western immunological approaches, this would indicate a need for diversification. A more inclusive curriculum would include studies that look at gender-specific immunological responses, or that include research carried out in different socio-cultural contexts. Integrating patient case studies from various ethnic backgrounds can also offer students an opportunity to explore how immunological diseases manifest and are treated in different communities, fostering a more comprehensive understanding of the field.

The pedagogical approaches employed should be varied to cater to diverse learning styles. While lectures might form the backbone of the module, these could be supplemented with other teaching methods. For example, lab sessions could give students hands-on experience in immunological techniques, while group discussions could encourage peer-to-peer learning. We might also consider guest lectures from experts who can bring different cultural or disciplinary perspectives into the classroom. These varied approaches are not just inclusive; they also serve to deepen students' understanding by engaging them through different modes of learning.

Assessment is another important area where EDI can be incorporated meaningfully. Written exams are often the default form of assessment, but they may not be the most equitable way to evaluate all students. Students for whom English is not their first language, or who have specific learning needs, might find written exams particularly challenging. It would therefore be beneficial to include a range of assessment methods. Oral presentations can help students develop public speaking skills and offer a different medium through which they can express their understanding. Portfolio submissions could allow for a more nuanced representation of a student's skills and understanding, capturing their progress over the course of the module. Peer assessments for group projects can also provide valuable insights into teamwork and collective problem-solving, skills that are vital in the clinical setting.

Creating a classroom environment where all students feel seen and heard is perhaps the most intangible yet vital aspect of integrating EDI. This could be facilitated through open forums or dedicated sessions where the class can discuss the importance of diversity and inclusion in clinical practice and research. Such conversations give students the vocabulary and the conceptual framework to think about these issues critically. Furthermore, allowing space for students to share personal experiences or perspectives can enrich the collective understanding and make for a more inclusive learning environment.

Curriculum design checklist

Content

- Review existing course materials to identify any gaps or biases.
- Incorporate research and case studies from diverse geographic and cultural contexts.
- Include gender-specific and LGBTQ+ relevant immunological studies.
- Add patient case studies representing various ethnic and socio-economic backgrounds.

Teaching methodology

- Audit current teaching methods to assess their inclusivity.
- Introduce a blend of pedagogical approaches such as lectures, labs, and interactive discussions.
- Invite guest speakers from diverse backgrounds and specialisms.
- Implement active learning techniques to engage various learning styles.

Assessment techniques

- Evaluate the fairness and inclusivity of existing assessment methods.
- Introduce multiple forms of assessment (e.g., written exams, oral presentations, portfolios).
- Include peer assessments for group work to evaluate teamwork and collaboration skills.
- Provide options for alternative assessments for students with specific learning needs.

Classroom culture

- Create an EDI statement for the course syllabus that outlines your commitment to these principles.
- Allocate time in the schedule for open discussions about EDI issues in clinical immunology.

- Establish a mechanism for anonymous feedback regarding EDI concerns within the course.
- Foster an environment where students are encouraged to share diverse perspectives.

Continuous improvement

- Conduct mid-term and end-of-term evaluations focusing on EDI aspects of the course.
- Seek feedback from students and colleagues to identify areas for improvement.
- Regularly update course materials to include the latest diverse perspectives and research.
- Review and adjust the course annually to align with evolving EDI best practices.

Conclusion

It is clear that the design of a biomedical science degree requires a thoughtful approach that accommodates the diverse needs and aspirations of its student body. This is essential for preparing students not only for successful careers in biomedical science, but also for roles in various related fields. The curriculum must be robust, relevant, and reflective of real-world biomedical science applications, ensuring that students gain both the theoretical knowledge and practical skills necessary for their future careers.

The curriculum should be continually reviewed and updated to remain current with the advances in biomedical technology and the evolving landscape of healthcare. Regular consultation with industry professionals, inclusion of diverse perspectives, and adherence to the latest educational and professional standards ensure that the curriculum remains relevant and effective.

At the heart of a well-designed biomedical science degree is the commitment to producing graduates who are competent, ethical, and adaptable, capable of navigating the complexities of the biomedical field. As educators, our role is to provide a curriculum that not only imparts knowledge and skills but also inspires a lifelong passion for learning and discovery in our students. By doing so, we contribute to the shaping of future professionals who are equipped to make significant contributions to biomedical science and healthcare.

References

1. Lisko SA, O'Dell V. Integration of Theory and Practice: Experiential Learning Theory and Nursing Education. *Nurs Educ Perspect.* 2010;31(2):106–108.
2. McTighe J, Wiggins G. *Understanding by Design Framework*. Association for Supervision and Curriculum Development. Published online 2012. https://www.sabes.org/sites/default/files/news/5_UbD_WhitePaper0312%5B1%5D.pdf
3. Felder RM, Brent R. Understanding Student Differences. *J Eng Educ.* 2005;94(1):57–72.
4. Prince M Does Active Learning Work? A Review of the Research. *J Eng Educ.* 2004;93(3):223–231.

5. Lee Olson C, Kroeger KR. Global Competency and Intercultural Sensitivity. *J Studies Int Educ.* 2001;5(2):116–137.

6. Harden RM. AMEE Guide No. 21: Curriculum Mapping: A Tool for Transparent and Authentic Teaching and Learning. *Med Teach.* 2001;23(2):123–137.

7. Grant J Principles of curriculum design. In: Swanwick, Tim, Forrest, Kirsty, O'Brien, Bridget C. (Eds.) *Understanding Medical Education.* John Wiley & Sons, Ltd; 2018:71–88.

8. Biggs J Constructive Alignment in University Teaching. *HERDSA Rev High Educ.* 2014;1: 5–22. Published online 2014.

9. Herreid CF. *Start with a Story: The Case Study Method of Teaching College Science.* NSTA Press; 2007.

10. Fink LD. The Power of Course Design to Increase Student Engagement and Learning. *Peer Rev.* 2007;9(1):13–17.

11. Mansilla VB, Duraising ED. Targeted Assessment of Students' Interdisciplinary Work: An Empirically Grounded Framework Proposed. *J Higher Educ.* 2007;78(2):215–237.

12. Espinosa LL, Turk JM, Taylor M, Chessman HM. Race and Ethnicity in Higher Education: A Status Report. Published online 2019. Accessed May 4, 2023. https://vtechworks.lib.vt.edu/handle/10919/89187

13. Smith DG. *Diversity's Promise for Higher Education: Making It Work.* JHU Press; 2020.

14. Chen A Addressing Diversity on College Campuses: Changing Expectations and Practices in Instructional Leadership. *High Educ Stud.* 2017;7(2):17.

15. Young K, Punnett A, Suleman S. A Little Hurts a Lot: Exploring the Impact of Microaggressions in Pediatric Medical Education. *Pediatrics.* 2020;146(1). doi:10.1542/peds.2020-1636

16. Welkener MM. The Skillful Teacher: On Technique, Trust, and Responsiveness in the Classroom. *J Higher Educ.* 2008;79(5):610–612.

17. Amechi MH, Estera A. Student Engagement in Higher Education: Theoretical Perspectives and Practical Approaches for Diverse Populations ed. by Stephen J. Quaye and Shaun R. Harper (review). *The Rev High Educ.* 2017;40(3): 473–475.

18. Bridgstock R, Grant-Iramu M, McAlpine A. Integrating Career Development Learning into the Curriculum: Collaboration with the Careers Service for Employ-ability. *J Teach Learn Grad Employab.* 2019;10(1):56–72.

19. Lisá E, Hennelová K, Newman D. Comparison between Employers' and Students' Expectations in Respect of Employability Skills of University Graduates. *Int J Work-Integrated Learnin.* 2019;20(1):71–82.

20. Quinlan KM, Renninger KA. Rethinking Employability: How Students Build on Interest in a Subject to Plan a Career. *High Educ.* 2022;84(4):863–883.

21. Badoer E, Hollings Y, Chester A. Professional Networking for Undergraduate Students: A Scaffolded Approach. *J Further High Educ.* 2021;45(2):197–210.

22. QAA. UK Quality Code for Higher Education. Part A: Setting and Maintaining Academic Standards. *The Frameworks for Higher Education Qualifications of UK Degree-Awarding Bodies, Quality Assurance Agency for Higher Education Glouces-ter,* 2019.

23. IBMS. *Criteria and Requirements for the Accreditation of MSc Degrees in Biomedical Science;* 2020.

24. IBMS. *Criteria and Requirements for the Accreditation of BSc (Hons) Degrees in Biomedical Science;* 2020.

25. The Quality Assurance Agency for Higher Education. *Subject Benchmark Statement Biomedical Sciences,* 2023.

2 Practitioner involvement

Alex Liversidge and Helen Battersby

The pathway from practitioner to academic

In the United Kingdom, Healthcare Scientists occupy a unique and integral role within the healthcare system. This is largely due to their comprehensive training, which combines academic rigour with professional expertise. Upon completing their educational programmes, these professionals are well-prepared to enter the workforce. However, qualification is not the end of their professional journey; rather, it serves as a springboard for a career that is both dynamic and continually evolving.

As they gain experience and expertise, Healthcare Scientists often find themselves at a crossroads, facing several divergent career pathways. One such avenue is the managerial or leadership pathway. Professionals who venture down this route often ascend to roles that demand strategic acumen, team leadership, and administrative oversight. These roles may involve responsibilities such as budget management, staffing decisions, and policy formulation. While this pathway offers the opportunity to enact systemic change and influence the broader healthcare landscape, it also comes with its own set of challenges, including a high level of responsibility and a skill set that extends beyond mere scientific expertise.

Another common trajectory is the clinical pathway. Healthcare Scientists who opt for this route are deeply embedded in the realms of patient care, diagnostics, and treatment planning. Their work is often on the cutting edge of medical science, using the latest technologies and methodologies to improve patient outcomes. This pathway allows for a specialised focus on scientific research and application but also requires strong interpersonal skills for effective collaboration with patients and other healthcare professionals.

A third option is the quality management pathway, which is particularly suited for those with a meticulous eye for detail and an unwavering commitment to upholding high standards of care. Professionals in this field are often responsible for auditing clinical practices, implementing quality control measures, and ensuring compliance with various regulatory frameworks. Their work is not only crucial for the continuous improvement of healthcare services but also instrumental in maintaining public trust in the healthcare system.

DOI: 10.4324/9781003383994-4

Lastly, some Healthcare Scientists find their calling in the training pathway. These individuals often possess a natural aptitude for pedagogy and choose to focus on educating the next generation of healthcare professionals. Whether through academic lecturing, clinical training, or the development of educational programmes, their work ensures that future Healthcare Scientists are as well-prepared as possible to meet the challenges and opportunities of this multifaceted profession.

What can practitioners bring to curriculum design?

The design of the content of the modules should follow both a process[1] and a content model of curriculum[2]. The content model is concerned with what students learn, and the transmission of subject knowledge from subject experts (the practitioner) to new students. These are the facts which are introduced early in the students' journey and the areas covered tend to be influenced or dictated by accrediting criteria. The process model, however, looks at students as active participants in the construction of this knowledge and in the development of understanding. It is easy to follow an objective-based approach[3] (learning outcomes) used throughout higher education (HE) when familiar with the vocational training methods used in practice such as the IBMS Registration Portfolio[4] which also follows this method.

We can provide the theoretical knowledge (content) required to understand the subject in the scheduled lectures followed by short revision questions and/or online activities to test student comprehension week-by-week. The practical sessions associated with the modules then apply this knowledge by testing 'patient' samples and analysing the results. Where possible, these sessions should use the modern technology and techniques used in a pathology laboratory setting to mimic real-life work. Quality control and quality assurance should be incorporated into tutorials where the interpretation of these results, together with the practice analysis of dummy patient pathology results, is discussed. The combination of this approach equips the students with the understanding of the subject in a pathology laboratory context which they then apply in the assessment setting using a case study scenario[5]. This strategy clearly follows Bloom's taxonomy[6] where the student moves through the six levels of learning from the simple to the complex, assimilating their knowledge through application and analysis, evaluation, and finally synthesis. It is important to think about a recent graduate employability skills survey conducted on behalf of IBMS here: encourage the students to think outside of one particular discipline when suggesting further testing, for example, a Haematology module including Biochemistry tests for haematinics if the patient results suggest anaemia[7]. The students respond positively to these types of analysis since they tend to be medical 'puzzles' rather than requiring rote regurgitation of facts. The disadvantage of case study-type exercises is that often there is no 'correct' answer which can cause anxiety - encourage the students to justify their diagnoses and explain their reasoning for requesting further investigations. This is reflective of life as a Healthcare Scientist especially when working alone on a shift and so encourages autonomous thinking, and confidence in their decision-making skills but an awareness of the responsibility this brings. The outcome of this approach can be judged by two internal measures: results of assessments and student satisfaction, but it should also improve the employability skills of graduates and therefore improve a Key Performance Indicator (KPI) for student outcomes.

Basing the module content around a real-world context is something practitioners are uniquely placed to do, an approach we should be keen to do because we 'showcase' the role. Most students choosing this degree have an element of curiosity in the medical field and so illustrating the theory with authentic activities throughout such as anonymised case studies, keeps their interest and offers them a tangible connection to the subject matter. This strategy has been positively received, as evidenced by student feedback and has led to several requests for placements. Of course, practitioners have a wealth of experience to generate exemplar results for a variety of conditions they have investigated during their careers.

Practitioners are also a valuable resource when educating students about the accreditation of their degree and what this means in terms of employability. While careers departments are able to offer general guidance, practitioners possess the nuanced understanding needed to explain what it means in the context of specific job markets. They can advise students on how to highlight this important credential on job applications, especially since potential employers may not be familiar with the accreditation status of various Higher Education Institutions (HEIs). They can also guide students through the maze of career pathways that degree accreditation can open up. Their first-hand experience in the field makes them uniquely qualified to introduce students to relevant regulatory and professional bodies, as well as to the processes required for various career trajectories. This level of detail and personal insight is something that traditional careers departments may struggle to provide, making practitioners an indispensable asset in the design and implementation of a robust, relevant curriculum.

What can practitioners bring to assessment design?

The involvement of practitioners with curriculum design to accurately reflect the knowledge and skills needed to work within a biomedical or pathology discipline naturally leads to practitioners creating assessments for students. In keeping with pedagogical practice, teaching, learning, and assessment should be 'constructively aligned'[8], and as such, if practitioners are involved in curriculum design and content then they must also play an active role in the assessment design.

Case studies for assessment

In the design of assessments, practitioners bring a level of authenticity and real-world applicability that is difficult to replicate through purely academic means. Given that the curriculum often employs real-life case studies to facilitate the transfer of knowledge, it stands to reason that summative assessments should mirror these real-world scenarios[5]. Practitioners, with their hands-on experience in the field, can craft case studies for assessments that are not only authentic but also highly relevant to the challenges students may face in their future roles.

Case studies as a means of assessment demonstrate authenticity and validity by their use of 'real-life' situations[5], with an approach that is highly applicable to working as a healthcare scientist. They are an opportunity to evaluate a range of skills, knowledge and understanding within a single assessment, while covering the depth of a module as a whole. They are also ideal for incorporating into summative assessment, not only can it test a student's knowledge around the specific topic, but also how successfully they can apply that knowledge to a clinical situation.

This not only cements the skills necessary to perform many healthcare scientist roles, but so too, many other duties seen in a wide range of science graduate positions. The Criteria and Requirements for the Accreditation of BSc (Hons) Degrees in Biomedical Science set out by the IBMS require that assessments are authentic[9]. Therefore, direct involvement from Healthcare Scientists, particularly in clinical modules, helps to ensure this authenticity. Healthcare Scientists who are also academics are uniquely positioned to infuse assessments with insights into current clinical practices, laboratory techniques, and professional standards. Their contributions enable students to better understand how academic theory translates into clinical practice, thereby enriching their own academic and professional development.

How assessment can develop graduate skills and attributes

Competition for trainee healthcare scientist positions is fierce, and the opportunities to gain a position are limited, therefore many employers looking to recruit recent graduates will often deploy a case study exercise or questions based on real-life scenarios as part of the interview process. This can be seen particularly in the recruitment to large, annual training programmes such as the NSHC STP which deploys a range of interview techniques to filter and assess candidates including a situational judgement test[10]. While theoretical knowledge of a specific discipline is important, employers are seeking to identify those graduates with key skills and attributes to make certain they employ the best candidate for the role. This helps to ensure that new employees already possess or can quickly gain the skills required for the role and potentially limits a high turnover of staff, which is critical in a highly specialised and demanding healthcare setting. Employers in these scenarios are seeking to evaluate a candidate's ability to display the core skills and attributes of a Healthcare Scientist. Typically, these case study exercises in an interview situation not only assess the candidate's knowledge but can also include evaluation of their data analysis, critical reasoning, and decision-making skills. By having academic Healthcare

Scientists embedded into the teaching and curriculum assessment design to provide authenticity, we are providing students with an opportunity to learn and be formatively assessed using this style. Therefore, the experience of case studies as part of an assessment such as an exam could translate to the interview situation. Students can be more confident that they have had already gained substantial experience of this process previously in summative assessment situations and are likely to be more adept at demonstrating their knowledge and skill set. In addition, given that we are able to build in elements to assessments that are specific to practising as a Healthcare Scientist, such as scope of practice, this can offer students key insights and provide a unique skill that other candidates may not possess.

The training and development of many clinical practitioners in a variety of roles in healthcare and biomedical science often follow rigorous training schemes or as discussed, in creation of detailed portfolios. These schemes often have inbuilt assessments for trainees to primarily ensure they have sufficient knowledge and skills expertise to achieve Health and Social Care Professions Council (HCPC) registration status. They include internal assessment of a trainee's ability to perform certain laboratory functions to assist with the day-to-day processing and analysis of samples. Or they can also include more formal assessment methods such as the Independent Assessment of Clinical Competence (IACC) to assess the readiness of trainees to practise as a newly qualified, threshold entry Clinical Scientist[11] or the completion and assessment of the IBMS portfolio[4]. The IBMS states that the 'IBMS Registration Training Portfolio is a record of evidence showing that candidates have achieved the competencies and standards outlined in the Registration Training Portfolio and meet the HCPC standards of proficiency'. Healthcare Scientist trainees therefore are assessed on both their appropriateness and capability by actively presenting the scenarios in which they have applied their scientific knowledge and skills, together with a wider consideration of the context of their work and self-reflection. Indeed, in the IACC, Clinical Scientist trainees are given a range of case-based discussions that reflect the typical clinical scenarios of a Clinical Scientist which they must analyse and interpret. Therefore, students enrolled on biomedical science undergraduate degree courses that directly feed into Healthcare Science professions can only benefit from aligning their module assessments to those they are likely to encounter within a professional setting. Having practitioners involved in the development and design of these assessments provides a wider context of testing. Practitioners are able to incorporate elements that reflect unique and specific aspects of the role of a Healthcare Scientist, for example, scope of practice and NHS pathways.

After registration has been completed, ongoing regular assessment to demonstrate further application of their knowledge, skills maintenance and competency is a necessary requirement for all laboratory staff including healthcare scientists. Accreditation inspections of diagnostic laboratories by regulatory agencies such as the United Kingdom Accreditation Service (UKAS)[12] and Medicines and Healthcare products Regulatory Agency (MHRA)[13,14] and the

IBMS[15] occur regularly to perform a safety audit of the laboratory's operations and conditions. Part of this audit procedure is to assess and encourage reliable assessment of the training and competency of scientific and laboratory staff in their roles and skills. Therefore, having assessment(s) during their time as undergraduates that closely reflects the type of assessment that is carried out in the professional setting can help the student to demonstrate skills and knowledge at both the recruitment stage and to be prepared for their professional role.

Employability & graduate jobs

Why is it important that we get the course content right?

The Government White Paper: Skills for Jobs[16] has clearly identified a skills gap which impacts the country economically. It is stated that there are not enough healthcare professionals, which we have first-hand experience of in practice. It can be difficult for NHS trusts to recruit graduates as an IBMS-accredited degree is the only approved method of becoming a Biomedical Scientist. Without an accredited degree, graduates are only able to apply for unqualified grade roles and have to complete top-up modules in order to fill in any gaps between their degree and an accredited one. Universities and NHS trusts can work together to identify needs and feed these into curriculum design for the process of accreditation thus, the situation can be improved for these large employers, usually situated near universities in urban areas, by improving the quality of the degree courses offered through accreditation. This is also important when competing with other local HEIs, especially since the interest in STEM courses is expected to increase after the Covid-19 pandemic as it has become apparent that they are a better investment for the student, society, and the economy. Healthcare Scientists also have clear career pathways set by their respective accrediting and regulatory bodies; it is our responsibility to ensure that pathway is clearly communicated to the students. Preferably this should take place prior to enrolment, through the development of school and college outreach and liaison exercises, so that students enrol on the correct degree in the first instance. After they have started their degree, there should be regular support provided for their development of professional skills. Practitioners can directly help in these aspects, for example, by contributing to a 'Professional Scientific Practice' type module where graduate skills are developed, and vocational career pathways explained. Embedding Healthcare scientists into the academic teaching team on biomedical science courses also provides further unique opportunities for a student's career development. Practitioners are able to offer insight and highlight opportunities for students seeking employment within the NHS or acceptance to specific training schemes a route in which to make contact and network with departments and individual professionals directly. They are able to arrange events such as 'speed networking with a scientist' for students to be able to meet with a diverse range of NHS Healthcare Scientists, calling on their own professional networks to invite key individuals. Activities such as these allow students an opportunity to ask pertinent questions and increase their knowledge of the roles available to them. This is helpful not only for their career choices, but also allows them to create their own professional network before they have graduated. Work experience within all facets of the NHS is either severely restricted or prohibited, meaning that there is no access for many students prior to graduation. For those students who have shown interest and proactivity at these different events, they can build contacts that may enable them to gain access to assistance with job applications, with many students receiving feedback on their applications and even an alert to a potential vacancy within a department.

Improving the ability of students to apply for professional healthcare positions feeds directly into one of the KPIs often stated in HEI's Education Strategies: students' employment upon graduation. These strategies are developed from The Government's Department for Education (DfE) policy statements which are specifically looking at measures such as improving the quality of student outcomes[17]. As the Skills for Jobs white paper states, as a country we seem to be 'efficient at producing graduates, but less able to help people get the quality technical skills that employers want'. The Office for Students formalised these indicators in a consultation in 2022 which included a series of minimum standards, which every course in every university should be expected to achieve[18]. Universities whose outcomes fall below these minimum standards may then be given a notice to improve. If improvements are not made, fines could be levied, courses withdrawn, and ultimately, degree-awarding powers could be withdrawn. Therefore, good quality, accredited courses, developed with the aid of practitioners' experience, which progress to highly skilled professional posts upon graduation should be a clear aim of the HEI as well as the enrolling student.

The recent IBMS survey stated that 93% of responding employers believe that new graduates do not meet the requirements for qualified or trainee Biomedical Scientist interview[7]. This included skills deficiency in the use of basic equipment such as digital pipettes, a sound basic understanding of laboratory results and ideas for further testing or potential diagnoses, and experience in an NHS laboratory. Employers felt overstretched with the volume of training, stating that new and inexperienced graduates can impact on the development of existing staff. Another important aspect of laboratory work which can be overlooked in academic qualifications is quality management. It is increasingly important to embed the concept of quality from an early stage so that the graduate is aware that it is equally their responsibility within a team of professionals to incorporate quality in all aspects of their work.

However, as current or recent practitioners, we know exactly what skills and knowledge are required to perform the role of Biomedical or Clinical Scientist in various disciplines. It requires an ability to physically perform complex investigations and derive results but also to incorporate that information with clinical details and other test results to provide advice, diagnoses and treatment.

Practitioner support for accreditation

Degree accreditation is advantageous for several reasons. Firstly, it provides reassurance to prospective students that the quality of the course has been assessed independently and achieved a national benchmark for the subject. This affords the HEI a competitive edge for the market share of student enrolments. It also enables the graduate to pursue directly a specific career as a qualified Biomedical Scientist, which without an accredited degree will be more circuitous and costly (but not impossible). This directly benefits the student by increasing the career pathways options available upon graduation together with the employers who are able to recruit appropriately qualified personnel to their workforce.

The process of accrediting a degree with the IBMS may pose quite a challenge to a HEI, especially the first time they seek accreditation. The criteria for the content of an accredited BSc (Hons) Biomedical Science course may be prescriptive and clinically based, aspects of which may be missing from the history of more traditional academic staff[9]. This can be a shift away from what has traditionally been taught, sometimes over many years, on an existing Biomedical or Medical Science type course. Some of the accredited modules can be very specific to hospital pathology laboratories such as Transfusion Science as well. Although there may be some similarities with existing subject areas, often these new modules require input from additional members of staff with experience, and practitioners can be a relevant and timely source of knowledge here.

Practitioner support for placements

The development of a BSc Applied Biomedical Science route is an optional but invaluable pathway. It also requires accreditation by IBMS if the Registration Portfolio is to be completed during the placement through an IBMS-approved training laboratory[9]. Usually, the placement year is between Level 5 and Level 6 and thus changes the degree into an integrated, four-year course. Upon successful completion of the placement, degree, and verification of the Registration Portfolio, the student is awarded the IBMS Certificate of Competence[4] and is eligible to apply for registration as a Biomedical Scientist with the HCPC[19]. The advantages of this pathway are that the student completes their professional training prior to graduation and therefore does not need to search for trainee Biomedical Scientist roles upon graduation (which can be limited in numbers and very competitive). They are eligible to apply for qualified, Agenda for Change (AfC) Band 5 Biomedical Scientist posts immediately, and since the Registration Portfolio is generic in nature, this can be in any discipline and not limited to the department in which they completed their training. Positive aspects for the training laboratory are that they can use the placement as an extended probation period, to iron out any 'employability issues' prior to recruitment of the candidate into a permanent post. Both students and placement supervisors should use the opportunity to feedback to the HEI on aCny gaps in knowledge or skills which become apparent during the placement. This can in turn be used to demonstrate the relationship between local employer and HEI (required to maintain accreditation) and as a method of continual cycle of improvement of the HEI curriculum.

The drawbacks to placements are that they are most often in NHS pathology hospital settings, which tend to be unpaid and can lead to hardship for the student, especially if from a disadvantaged background. University bursaries may be available, but these are modest and tend not to cover the cost of living. Also, the burden for the training laboratory is high, students completing their second year of university may have little lab experience and not all relevant knowledge required and so may need more assistance than the average trainee Biomedical Scientist applicant. If there is a gap where the student needs to return to university to complete their final year, they may require a period of re-training or competency assessment once they have graduated. They may also not be successful when applying for qualified positions, there is no guarantee that a role is available at that time in the training laboratory, or the student may move location and seek employment elsewhere. There is also the issue of ambition, not all students may know what career they would like to pursue upon graduation, never mind which discipline they would like to work in. This is particularly true of the more specialist departments of larger pathology trusts and networks, which may only be referred to briefly in the course modules, are divided into different modules or are not covered at all.

To address the issue of lack of familiarity with hospital pathology laboratories working environments and the variety of disciplines found within, it may be pertinent to arrange a tour of each department for the students. However, this may not be easy to arrange, as these environments have restricted access for a variety of legitimate safety reasons and legal requirements and so needs to be formally arranged. With a large cohort of students, this can be time-consuming and physically difficult to accommodate. To ease the pressure on the laboratory staff, where possible the academic practitioner may be the one to conduct the tour, which enables them to pitch the information at the right level and link to areas of the course which are relevant (such as laboratory health and safety). This should also be useful for continual professional development (CPD) for the practitioner to be made aware of changes to practice which may require updates to the content of the course module(s). This maintains the currency and relevance of the module content.

The applied route accreditation process is facilitated by having a module lead who is/was a practitioner since they will be familiar with the route to qualification as a Biomedical Scientist. In their hospital role they may have supported candidates completing the Registration Portfolio directly or indirectly. In any case, there is a requirement for close collaboration with the participating laboratories as the accreditation criteria apply to both the HEI and placement laboratory. To facilitate the accreditation process, a gap analysis against the criteria should be performed with an action plan and evidence once each standard is achieved. On the HEI side, knowledge of the academic regulations and quality processes required to set up or make amendments to courses and pathways is also advantageous[20]. Usually, there is an existing placement department which can offer assistance, but it is worth being aware of the many personnel and health and safety requirements needed by both the NHS and HEI before students can be accepted into a hospital environment.

It is obvious that there needs to be a close relationship between the HEI and employers to facilitate the placement opportunities, which can be very competitive. However, the IBMS survey indicated that employer liaison committees, which should be an opportunity for placement hosts to feedback to the HEIs about their course content and any perceived lack of skills, do not tend to be well attended. Some commented that they seemed to be used solely for the benefit of HEIs and did little to help the employer. An alternative approach was to incorporate the employer liaison committee meeting into a training event for the placement staff. The agenda included updates to the undergraduate and postgraduate courses, re-accreditation news, and the opportunity for employers to feedback any graduate issues or suggestions for the courses. This was in turn relayed to the Course Directors and Head of Subject for consideration at a later course development event. There was an opportunity for any grade of staff in the placement laboratories who had an interest in supporting students through a Registration Portfolio and/or to verify candidate's work to attend this training to contribute towards their CPD. Because the HEI acknowledged the collaboration was invaluable, a lunch was provided which also improved attendance! Keeping a channel open between HEI and employers is vital, and the relationships that practitioners have built facilitates this, after all, most are training the next generation of Healthcare Scientists because they value their profession.

Support for professional qualifications

Practitioners have, by definition, completed their professional training in their chosen careers. Depending on their length in the post, they may have not followed the exact path that current students will be expected to complete, but they will have some experience of vocational training and assessment. It is usual for practitioners who enter academia to have had an element of training responsibility to their roles beforehand. Therefore, they may have direct or indirect experience in supporting trainee Healthcare Scientists through the registration process. The IBMS Registration Portfolio comprises vocational and specific practical elements which would be impossible (and inappropriate) to complete outside of an approved training laboratory (usually based in a hospital)[4]. However, there are several aspects of the knowledge segments of the more generic sections (such as personal responsibility and development, communication, equality & diversity and health & safety) which could be taught outside of the laboratory environment. Given that the training laboratories are under strain and this limits their ability to offer placement opportunities, there is scope for practitioners in academia to assist in delivering these areas. Perhaps assistance in this way may ease some of the burden that the training laboratories feel comes from the HEI when accepting placement students. An example of this is to provide online, recorded Registration Portfolio seminars which can be taught synchronously or viewed asynchronously around the students' schedules during the summer break prior to the placement starting in September. During these sessions there is an opportunity to discuss the Portfolio and verification process, each Portfolio module in detail and to set tasks to address some of the Portfolio knowledge requirements. Suggestions of tasks can also be made for the competence aspects which can complement or incorporate the training programmes set for each pathology department hosting the placement student. This seminar schedule does not need to be reserved only for those students due to commence a placement, the opportunity can be opened to others (those unable to financially accommodate another year in HE, or those unsuccessful in the placement application process, etc.) who wish to pursue a career as a Biomedical Scientist. Having a detailed knowledge of the portfolio structure and having some pieces of work completed already is invaluable for those graduates applying for Trainee Biomedical Scientist posts. It is a personal choice (and obviously depends upon workload, number of students, and other factors) as to whether the academic supporting these sessions is able to review the output of those attending but it is advisable to at least support those due to commence a placement. The academic review should demonstrate the feedback process through annotation and amendment as per the usual guidance from the IBMS but then signed off by the hospital training officer during the placement. It is helpful to also discuss what tasks are to be set with the hospital placement Training Managers to ensure they agree on their suitability.

When considering the direct pathway that a biomedical science course has to professional scientific roles in healthcare, it is clear that establishing links with those employed as such can only benefit the academic team supporting the students and the graduates themselves. This may be as a part-time or guest role within the HEI or as a permanent post, but there are mutual benefits also to the practitioner in supporting the development of the next generation of Healthcare Scientists through their involvement in academia.

Case study: Escape room revision aid

To incorporate case studies and a more realistic pathology laboratory workload together with acting as an autonomous professional in a light-hearted scenario, an escape room base formative assessment was created for a Transfusion Science module. It includes 'patient' results and covers several key topics from the module curriculum.

Revision aid introduction

You are a Biomedical Scientist working a night shift in a busy hospital lab. Several patients have been admitted acutely and the clinical staff are requesting that you help them. See if you can make it through the shift and keep everyone alive & well!

Revision aid tasks

Puzzle 1: A patient, Madison Rowan, is admitted through A&E and has been involved in a Road Traffic Collision (RTC). You receive a group and screen test. She is a 35-year-old woman who has had 3 previous pregnancies.

Puzzle 2: A little while later, the patient's red cell antibody screen result comes back positive. You set up an antibody panel and get the following pattern. Can you determine which antibody they have?

Puzzle 3: Finally, the Group & Screen is complete. You can put your feet up and have a brew. Just as you put the cup to your mouth the emergency bleep sounds. It's A&E, the patient is bleeding and requires some blood and components. What blood do you crossmatch?

Puzzle 4: Because this is a massive haemorrhage situation, the patient also requires some other blood components. Which of the following may be useful in this situation?

Puzzle 5: You ring A&E to inform them the additional blood components are ready. A porter arrives to pick up some blood. He's a bit unsure because the components are labelled Madison Rowan, but he's been told the patient is called Rowan Madison and the hospital ID number doesn't match. What do you do?

Puzzle 6: Which of the following alternatives to transfusion would probably help in this situation?

Puzzle 7: The patient is successfully operated on and the bleeding stops. She is moved to a ward where she is given some more blood, FFP and platelets. After a few hours the clinical staff notice that her oxygen saturation has decreased, and her blood pressure is very high. Her temperature is normal. What is the most likely serious adverse reaction in this situation?

Puzzle 8: The patient is extremely grateful for the care she has received and would like to become a blood donor when she fully recovers. Would this be possible?

Finally, the day shift staff appear, and you are free to go home.
YOU HAVE ESCAPED THE LAB!

Well done.

Disclaimer: Although possible, it is incredibly unlikely that a BMS would experience all of these situations in one shift. Equally, it is unlikely that a patient would experience all these clinical situations. It is a revision guide only, and no resemblance to real life should be inferred. Thanks for taking part, I hope it was useful.

This task is a fun way of testing the key learning outcomes for the Transfusion Science module such as interpreting blood groups and investigating antibody identification panels which are core skills for this pathology discipline. Feedback for the module overall and the activity is good, with the resources supplied to test understanding such as the revision aid above in particular rated highly.

Conclusion

The involvement of practitioners in a biomedical science degree program is an indispensable element in bridging the gap between academic theory and real-world practice. Their direct engagement in the curriculum and assessment design enriches the educational experience by providing students with a deep, practical understanding of the biomedical science field. This approach ensures that the course content is not only academically sound but also resonates with the current demands and advancements in biomedical science. Practitioners bring to the table a wealth of professional experience, technical skills, and industry insights, making them uniquely qualified to guide students through the complexities of biomedical science. Their contribution to the curriculum includes the integration of case studies, practical scenarios, and hands-on experiences, which are instrumental in preparing students for the challenges they will face as future professionals. This hands-on, experiential learning approach is crucial for developing critical thinking, analytical skills, and the ability to apply theoretical knowledge in practical situations.

Beyond curriculum design, practitioners also play a crucial role in mentoring students, providing career guidance, and offering insights into the various pathways and opportunities within the biomedical science field. Their first-hand experience and knowledge are invaluable in helping students navigate their career choices, understand the requirements for professional qualifications, and make informed decisions about their future.

Overall, practitioner involvement in biomedical science education is essential for creating a comprehensive, relevant, and dynamic learning experience. It aligns academic learning with industry standards and expectations, thereby ensuring that graduates are well-equipped, not just academically, but also with the practical skills and knowledge required to excel in the ever-evolving field of biomedical science.

References

1. Stenhouse L. *An Introduction to Curriculum Research and Development.* Heinemann, 1975.
2. Hirst PK. *Knowledge and the curriculum. A collection of Philosophical Papers.* Routledge and Kegan Paul, 1974.
3. Tyler RW. *Basic Principles of Curriculum and Instruction.* University of Chicago Press, 1949.
4. Institute of Biomedical Science. *Registration Training Portfolio 4th edition (V4.3)*, 2022. https://www.ibms.org/education/registration-portfolio/
5. Cox S. *Case Studies for Active Learning. HEA: Hospitality, Leisure, Sport and Tourism Network*, 2009. https://www.heacademy.ac.uk/node/3868
6. Bloom BS, Engelhart MD, Furst EJ, Hill WH, Krathwohl DR. (1956). Taxonomy of educational objectives: The classification of educational goals. In: Bloom, B.S. (Ed.) *Handbook I: Cognitive Domain.* David McKay Company.
7. Hussain T, Hicks M *Assessing Employability Skills.* The Biomedical Scientist p18–22, 2022. https://www.thebiomedicalscientist.net/science/assessing-employability-skills
8. Biggs JB, Tang, C. *Teaching for Quality Learning at University* (4th ed.). Open University Press, 2011.
9. Institute of Biomedical Science (2021) *Criteria and Requirements for the Accreditation of BSc (Hons) Degrees in Biomedical Science September 2022 – July 20232 V2.1.* https://www.ibms.org/resources/documents/criteria-and-requirements-for-the-accreditation-and-re/
10. National School of Healthcare Science *Scientist Training Programme*, 2023. https://nshcs.hee.nhs.uk/programmes/stp/
11. National School of Healthcare Science *Independent Assessment of Clinical Competence*, 2023. https://nshcs.hee.nhs.uk/programmes/stp/trainees/independent-assessment-of-clinical-competence-iacc/
12. United Kingdom Accreditation Service *Medical Laboratories – Requirements for Quality and Competence.* ISO Standards 15189:2022, 2022. https://www.ukas.com/accreditation/standards/medical-laboratory-accreditation/
13. Medicines and Healthcare Products Regulatory Agency *Blood: authorisations and safety reporting*, 2014. https://www.gov.uk/guidance/blood-authorisations-and-safety-reporting
14. UK Government *The Blood Safety and Quality Regulations -SI 2005/50*, 2005. https://www.legislation.gov.uk/uksi/2005/50/contents/made
15. Institute of Biomedical Science *Clinical Laboratory Standards for Qualification*, 2018. https://www.ibms.org/resources/documents/ibms-laboratory-training-standards/
16. UK Government. *Skills for Jobs: Lifelong Learning for Opportunity and Growth.* Crown, 2021. https://www.gov.uk/government/publications/skills-for-jobs-lifelong-learning-for-opportunity-and-growth
17. UK Government, Department for Education *Higher education policy statement & reform consultation.* Crown, 2022. https://assets.publishing.service.gov.uk/government/uploads/system/uploads/attachment_data/file/1057091/HE_reform_command-paper-web_version.pdf
18. UK Government, Office for Students *Consultation on a new approach to regulating student outcomes.* Crown, 2022. https://www.officeforstudents.org.uk/media/c46cb18a-7826-4ed9-9739-1e785e24519a/consultation-on-a-new-approach-to-regulating-student-outcomes-ofs-2022-01.pdf

19. Health & Care Professions Council *Registration*, 2023. https://www.hcpc-uk.org/registration/
20. LBU Academic Regulations 2020–21 *Section 13: Approval, Validation, Monitoring and Review*. https://www.leedsbeckett.ac.uk/-/media/files/our-university/academic-regulations/full-current-academic-regulations/academic-regulations-202021.pdf

Part II
Teaching methodologies

3 Research-integrated teaching

Ismini Nakouti and Donna Johnson

What is research-integrated teaching and why is it important?

Biomedical science is a swift-moving research area. With the widespread use of next-generation and newer sequencing technologies, as well as rapid developments in subjects such as innovative gene-editing, cancer immunotherapy and stem-cell technology, scientific innovations in health care have been coming faster and faster across the field. Globally more than $240 billion is invested in health research per year with the US and China being the major leaders[1]. The insights of this research should be integrated into teaching by academics[2].

In 2005 Healey[3] described the relationship between teaching and research and divided it into two separate elements: One extends from 'student as audience' (teacher lead) to 'student as participant' (student lead) and the second extends from 'emphasis on research content' to 'emphasis on research processes and problems'[3]. Research-intergraded teaching in Higher Education is an area that has attracted a lot of attention. It is not a new concept as it goes back to 1990[4].

It is important to communicate to the students revolutionary developments in biomedical science as it challenges them to develop essential skills, such as critical thinking, multiple problem solving, and to develop further new technology. These fundamental cognitive skills should evolve from the early days of their education and continue throughout their academic life. Embedding research in undergraduate teaching is showing students that science is multiplex and under debate. Universities have the responsibility to demonstrate that the scientific world is continuously progressing by research.

Very often research and teaching are regarded as two completely different activities. This appears to be a myth. Research focuses on attracting external funding, submitting manuscripts, and collaborating with the NHS, industry, or various research institutions. Teaching involves student contact hours, curriculum development, learning outcomes, marking, and administration[5]. However, the relationship between teaching and research should be symbiotic and research should be integrated with the curriculum of the biomedical science programmes.

DOI: 10.4324/9781003383994-6

Research has always been a major part of the biomedical science curriculum but recently there has been a trend (and pressure) to integrate essential research elements into teaching. However, it is wrong to assume that all good academics are good researchers and vice versa. There are a great number of institutions around the world where a vast number of staff are non-research active. Most practitioners don't even have a PhD. Also, research-based teaching very often is limited to staff who are successful in obtaining research money internally or externally, with limited time for undergraduate teaching. Funding is highly concentrated. Should teaching be driving research funding allocation?

Challenges

There is no denying the benefits of research-integrated teaching, however, it does come with some challenges. Primarily we must get the 'integrated' right. We need to ensure that we have the basics in place so students are able to understand the more complex ideas that often come with research. This leads to pitching the content at the right level, we would likely talk about research in slightly different ways depending on the level we're teaching at. Finally, we need to make sure that whatever research we talk about is strongly and explicitly linked with the wider teaching concepts covered in a module.

Biomedical science degrees are generally set up so that each sub-discipline covers more complicated ideas as students progress through the levels and we need to follow along with this when we bring real-world research into our modules. While at level four we are going to be concentrating on getting the fundamental skills and knowledge in place, bringing in examples of actual research is a really good way of setting the context for the topics and so scaffolds student learning, for example, we can use topics like disease epidemiology to introduce basic maths skills (powers of ten, percentages etc). Setting context early and then reinforcing it as students move through their degree is key, having a context in which to place their knowledge is going to help with understanding the relevance of what they're learning and increase motivation and engagement.

Integrating research gets slightly easier as we progress to levels five and six. Here students are learning about more specific topics within the sub-disciplines so it is relatively easier to identify relevant research to talk about, we may even be able to draw from our own research. The biggest problem here is going to be how we communicate the more complex ideas in ways that do not overwhelm the students and how to link them with the more straightforward concepts we may be trying to teach.

One of the larger challenges with research-integrated teaching is assessment. Assessing research-integrated teaching can be difficult because, depending on the type of assessment, there may not be a single completely right answer. If we are asking students to interpret data for example, then there may be multiple potential outcomes that are valid, even if there is a particular one we have in mind when writing the assessment.

There may be challenges with the time and knowledge needed to write research-integrated assessments. We need to consider the module ILO(s) and concept(s) we want to assess, then identify suitable material for inclusion in the assessment and this should be preceded by similar decisions about the taught content that feeds into the assessment. Identification or creation of suitable data for inclusion is particularly hampered if we are newer to a topic, it's not always straightforward to know what will work for what we want it for even as experts let alone topics we are less experienced with. This will be doubly true if we're looking at data in a clinical context without ever having worked in a clinical setting.

Research-integrated teaching can, undoubtedly, be significantly influenced by the size of the cohort. In smaller groups, the integration of research and teaching is a readily tangible educational strategy that can yield substantial positive results. Working with smaller cohorts provides us with the flexibility to foster an environment that is more responsive to individual student needs. Here, we can focus on developing a research-oriented mindset, and encourage students to question, rather than just absorb information. This is an approach that often mimics the iterative and explorative nature of actual scientific research, lending a practical edge to the learning experience. The staff–student interaction that smaller cohorts allow can greatly enhance the feedback process too. In such settings, feedback becomes a dialogue, a two-way process that enables students to better understand their strengths and weaknesses and offers us insights into our teaching effectiveness. This ongoing feedback mechanism is crucial in a research-oriented educational framework, mirroring the peer review process that is integral to scientific research. It's not just about the staff-student dynamics though. Smaller cohorts also cultivate an environment conducive to peer learning, a significant component in research-integrated teaching. Peer discussions and collaborations can stimulate critical thinking, promote the cross-fertilisation of ideas, and help students gain different perspectives on the same problem—a fundamental skill in any research endeavour.

Many of us teach large cohorts however and here the dynamics significantly shift. The ability to tailor teaching to individual needs is greatly diluted, providing personalised feedback becomes an uphill task, and the quality of peer interactions might also be compromised. In such scenarios, maintaining student engagement can be challenging, and some students might struggle to keep up with the pace of the course. This could potentially jeopardise their ability to fully grasp the complex interplay between research and learning, ultimately impacting the efficacy of research-integrated teaching.

Meeting the challenges

So how do we overcome these challenges in order to maximise the benefits we and our students can get from research-integrated teaching? In a perfect world, this would be approached as a team-based exercise at the course design stage. The best scenario is to have research integrated throughout a degree course and into all modules and this cannot be done effectively in isolation. Biomedical science teaching teams generally have multiple staff, each with a mix of expertise across the sub-disciplines, some will be research-active and some may not be but each will bring something unique and valuable to the table. As our courses get periodically reviewed, this is a good time to look at how we use research in our teaching and then build it in from the ground up. However, it is possible that we may be working to integrate research into individual modules. This will have positives and negatives—we can focus more on the specifics of what we want/need to include but we may not have the necessary knowledge to take full advantage nor are we able to develop links with other taught content that may be relevant. In this situation, it is good to look for support from other people teaching the module and those with more specific expertise, while they may not have time to produce or locate data, they will be able to point out suitable sources. For linking to other content, if we have a reasonable idea of what is being taught in relevant modules then we can signpost in our own sessions to these materials and try to develop these links for students to follow within those other modules.

In order to make assessment more straightforward and to identify where the best place is to integrate research it is important to define clear learning outcomes for a module. Here we can align ILOs to assessment and this has the added advantage of providing clarity to students and they can get a good picture of why research is being included and how, how it fits into the context of the module and the real-world applications of taught content, all things that are suggested to promote student engagement and a deeper learning approach.

For the assessment of research-integrated teaching, using an authentic assessment approach can be valuable. Authentic assessment is an approach to assessing learning that emphasises real-world tasks, situations and research data that students are likely to encounter outside of the classroom. In more traditional types of assessment, students tend to become more passive learners, prioritising memorisation of information rather than application. While remembering facts is useful, they can be quickly forgotten and information is more likely to be dealt with in isolation rather than through building links with other knowledge and experiences. By using authentic assessments with research-integrated teaching, students develop critical thinking and evaluation skills and are more engaged because the assessment type has more clearly defined links to their desired career paths and the real world. If we use assessment types such as paper analyses then we can embed similar activities in taught sessions to highlight the research and methods needed. In paper analyses, students are provided with a paper in advance of the assessment and then may be asked to interpret a figure/table or expand on an issue raised in the paper. In these types of questions, students should be giving an overview of what the figure shows and then link this to the conclusions made in the paper and provide supporting evidence from other research. Including a paper analysis also goes hand in hand with a session on how to read a paper that can easily be included in a research methods module and introduces them to activities they may encounter in journal clubs as well as giving them a good feel for the research. By using assessments like this, we then have the opportunity to include our own research or previously published research.

Perhaps the biggest challenge we need to overcome with research-integrated teaching is ensuring students are adequately prepared and supported. Depending on the level a module is set at, students may have very limited experience in reading about or handling research data, but research papers can feel particularly impenetrable for the experienced and inexperienced alike. We need to make sure that students are thoroughly introduced to the fundamentals of the research we want to use and then guided in how to use/interpret the data. We need to clearly communicate our expectations of them in terms of how the research should be used, especially if it forms a component of their assessment and we should be providing feedback throughout. More importantly, we need to clearly show the link between the research we are including and the topic we are teaching them.

When we are teaching larger cohorts we may need to restructure the learning environment to facilitate more intimate interactions. We could break the large class into smaller discussion groups who then work on specific problems. By creating these sub-units within a larger class, we can go some way to replicating the benefits of small cohort dynamics. Another potential solution is the integration of technology. Various platforms offer facilities that allow discussion forums and breakout rooms that can be harnessed to deliver a more individualised learning experience. For example, we can use online forums for students to share their research findings and provide peer feedback, stimulating active learning and critical thinking. Virtual labs can expose students to research methodologies and procedures, allowing them to experiment and learn in a risk-free environment and breakout rooms can facilitate focused group discussions or group work, promoting the kind of collaborative problem-solving integral to research.

The practice of integrating research into teaching, despite its inherent challenges, holds immense potential for transformative learning experiences, particularly within biomedical science. Research integration allows students to navigate the combination of theory and practice. Merging the investigative nature of research with classroom learning instils in students the skills necessary to challenge existing norms, developing them into active contributors to the scientific discourse rather than passive recipients of information. It can also help cultivate a sense of authenticity and relevance among learners. By engaging directly with ongoing research—whether through case studies, discussions on recent scientific papers, or even hands-on experimentation—students can better grasp the applicability and implications of what they learn. This, in turn, helps to enhance their motivation and engagement, both essential factors that influence academic success. The collaborative and interdisciplinary nature of research provides valuable lessons in teamwork, communication, and cross-disciplinary thinking. These soft skills, often underemphasised in traditional education models, are increasingly recognised as crucial for success in today's complex and interconnected world.

Another considerable advantage is the potential for personalisation. Research is seldom a one-size-fits-all endeavour. Similarly, research-integrated teaching can cater to diverse interests and career goals. For example, a student interested in genetic diseases might choose to delve into recent research on gene therapy, while another might focus on public health studies related to disease outbreaks. This freedom to explore areas of personal interest can lead to more profound learning experiences and increased student satisfaction.

Finally, research-integrated teaching can play a significant role in enhancing scientific literacy among our students—a crucial attribute in an age of information overload and 'fake news'. By engaging with research, students learn to scrutinise sources, evaluate evidence, and separate scientific facts from pseudoscience, which are critical skills both within and beyond the classroom.

Integrating research into teaching is not merely a beneficial pedagogical approach, but a necessity in the rapidly evolving field of biomedical science. By bridging the gap between theory and practice, fostering a sense of relevance and authenticity, nurturing critical soft skills, allowing personalisation of learning experiences, and enhancing scientific literacy, it promotes a holistic educational experience that adequately prepares students for the challenges of the future.

Case study 1: Genetics/genomics: Integrating publicly available research into teaching

Genetics and genomics, perhaps more so than any of the other sub-disciplines in biomedical science has seen a rapid series of advances, primarily off the back of the Human Genome Project and the associated development of technologies like next-generation sequencing. These advances have led to a significant shift in how this information is collected and used and this in turn has had a considerable impact on clinical practice. The increase in available genetic/genomic information has resulted in a greater degree of diagnostic/prognostic capability but has also brought with it a minefield of ethical and privacy concerns. It's not just the clinic when these advances have had an impact though, genetic/genomic technologies are widely integrated across multiple fields such as drug design, microbiology and public health.

It is increasingly difficult to separate the use of IT from genetics/genomics. The types and volumes of data produced, the analysis pipelines in place, and the need to access the repositories of data mean that anyone working in the field needs to have at least a reasonable understanding of using a computer. We are also faced with the need to interpret more complex data outputs, which brings with it a further need to be comfortable around computers and statistics.

These changes in the field mean that we need to think about what we teach our students and how. Genetics may be a very small component of a biomedical science degree but will have considerable relevance for most of the other sub-disciplines so we need to ensure that students not only have the basics in place but are also able to make the links between topics and modules.

A benefit of the advances and increased volume of publications along with the associated approach to data sharing means that we have access to a lot of freely available resources we can use to teach our students, often these are the same ones used in clinical practice. Sessions on genetics/genomics are ideal places to integrate published research into teaching:

- NCBI: Databases of information for SNPs, gene and protein sequences, BLAST searches and
- Varsome: Database for sequence info relating to mutations and diseases
- Ensembl: Databases of vertebrate genome information for SNPs, gene and protein sequences, BLAST searches and
- Galaxy: Web-based analysis program
- Nuffield Council on Bioethics: Repository of information on ethical issues associated with the life sciences

Publicly available research and data were embedded into two lectures covering aspects of genomics in the context of biotechnology and activities were designed to encourage students to engage in independent research to identify applications of the technologies.

The lectures in this level six biotechnology module centred around genomics are:

- The Genomic Revolution
    - This session covers the Human Genome Project and how the resulting technological advances have been applied to medicine
- Genome Editing
    - This session covers several methods for genome editing and their applications in medicine

Both of these topics are excellent starting points for integrating research. The sessions follow a similar format, there is a general introduction to the topic overall then we cover the methods/technologies in more detail. Following this we look at the applications of the technologies and finally there is consideration of the ethical implications (Table 3.1). Each general introduction is a story of how we got to the current state of the topic, what was the driving force behind the development of the earlier methods and who were the key drivers. Here we integrate earlier examples of research in the topics as a way of setting the scene and helping students to build a picture of how the flow of research results in an applied technology. More recent examples are then included with the current applications.

Independent research activities are set the week before a session and are discussed as a group at the end of each session.

The use of research in these sessions is designed to give students a better understanding of the application of cutting-edge technologies in medicine and

Table 3.1 Taught content

Section	Genomic revolution	Genome editing
Introduction	Research in the late 1800s-1980s, the importance of the Human Genome Project	Links to technologies covered in the Genomic revolution sessionDiscussion of early technologies and uses of editing
Methods	Next generation sequencing	Recombinant AAV, TALENS, CRISPR
Applications	Overview of NGS applications in cancer, infectious disease	Cystic fibrosis gene therapy, leukaemia therapies, production of isogenic cell lines
Ethics	Links to HGP ELSI and how this has impacted future research projects	Links to CRISPR babies, impact on field, more general consideration of ethical concerns around human genetic engineering
Independent activities	Personal genetic testing— would you get your genome sequenced? Why/why not?	'Outlandish' uses for genome editing

to become inspired by what is possible in this field. The independent study activities are designed to get students to apply a concept to themselves (personal genetics) and to help them think about a concept in related areas (uses for genome editing).

The biggest advantage of using research for teaching these topics is that there is so much of it available, and it is in a context that will have meaning for the students. It can be difficult to ensure that students fully understand the data used, especially when using SNP or sequencing data but detailed explanations are easily embedded in the sessions and there is a wealth of resources available to support this in their independent study. Such resources are also useful to staff as an aid to simplifying some of the more complex concepts covered.

Using research in these ways has led to good student outcomes, and their assessments generally show a deeper understanding of the topics. It has also led to some lively and interesting in-class discussions! As well as genetics/genomics, we can use this type of approach across multiple sub-disciplines. It is particularly useful for teaching immunology or cellular pathology for example, where we can use published research and data to build links between fundamental knowledge and its application in the clinic:

- Immunology: https://www.immunopaedia.org.za/clinical-cases/
- Cellular pathology: https://www.cellwiki.net/
- Haematology: https://www.hematologyinterest.com/case-studies.html
- Epidemiology: https://www.cdc.gov/training/epicasestudies/classroom.html

Case study 2: Microbiology (biofilms and antimicrobial resistance)

Antibiotic resistance is recognised as one of the greatest threats to global human health and modern medicine. The O'Neil Report on Antimicrobial Resistance, commissioned by the UK Government (PM: David Cameron) and Wellcome Trust, reported that by 2050, unless action is taken, the death toll due to antimicrobial-resistant strains can reach globally up to 10 million lives a year, which is equivalent to 1 person per every 3 seconds! Jim O'Neil is actually an economist, who warned that under the current scenario 300 million people will die due to antimicrobial resistance and the world is expected to sacrifice between 60 and 100 trillion USD if drug resistance is not addressed.

Biofilms-associated cells are well known to exhibit multiple drug resistance due to their unique characteristics, such as slow metabolic activity, polysaccharide production and persister cell formation to name a few. It is evident that cells enveloped in a biofilm are highly protected, which makes it difficult for antimicrobial agents to reach the living community. Moreover, cells attached to a biofilm demonstrate a lower growth rate than their planktonic (free-living) counterparts leading to decreased bacteriocidal action and therefore increased biofilm resistance[6].

This topic is a critical issue in biomedical science and emphasis needs to be highlighted to the students in order to understand the impact of antibiotic resistance and antimicrobial stewardship.

The pedagogic activity is embedded in the Microbiology Module attended by a large cohort of undergraduate students at level four. The goal is the transfer of research knowledge within the classroom environment. The focus is the formation and disruption of biofilms and their characteristics using a variety of intervention strategies, including antimicrobials. Emphasis is given to antimicrobial resistance and its impact on health care and our society. It addresses one of the most urgent subjects facing medicine today, the global spread of resistance mechanisms to the community. This session is designed to be a source used to explain to students the link between biofilms and antimicrobial resistance. The lecture also highlights the high risk of spreading multidrug resistant microorganisms to the community, health care services, and care homes.[19]

Approach

In order to access antimicrobial strategies a scientist needs to develop a suitable biofilm model. The students need to understand that development and problem-solving are directly linked to research. Also, very often development includes more than one model. During this session we demonstrate the different models and highlight the advantages and disadvantages, such as high throughput assays, small-scale technologies, time, cost, effectiveness, and training requirements. The audience appreciates that research is a multifactor concept where many aspects have to be considered. The next step includes the use of advanced technology to prove that the models support robust biofilms.

The theory behind SEM, atomic force and confocal microscopy is briefly explained. Most students at level four have experience with light microscopy in school but they haven't been exposed to more advanced techniques. It is very important for the students to understand that biofilms are morphologically heterogeneous and multilayered matrices, characteristics that contribute to their antimicrobial resistance. Microscopy is a powerful visual tool that helps students from different educational backgrounds to understand microbial structure. The students are able to understand microbial behaviour by examining 3D pictures of biofilms in the classroom, boosting conceptual learning. Visual tools encourage learners to become active participants and develop decision-making skills. They can process and analyse data quicker, which inspires them to become independent thinkers. It has been reported that first-year medical students favour visual learning, such as photographs and diagrams, over verbal. The study included subjects similar to biomedical science, such as Immunology, Genetics, and Microbiology[7].

The next step is to introduce high throughput scale-down sensor technology with the view to measuring antimicrobial efficacy and resistance against biofilms. High throughput screening is an established discipline in biomedical science, commonly used in research hospitals in the NHS. It allows the generation of large-scale data for medical analysis. The students are given a brief description of the research technique and are presented with a graph containing data from 96 small-scale experiments. They need to interpret them and identify areas of antimicrobial resistance. They appreciate how multiple antimicrobials can be tested against biofilms simultaneously with the design of a single experiment. Again, this process encourages students' conceptual learning. It encourages them to understand the theory and not just memorise the outcomes. This leads to a healthy debate in the classroom as to where these powerful tools can be used. How can we do things quicker and better in biomedical science?

Dynamic discussions also evolve around antimicrobial stewardship, which is the force to educate clinicians or pharmacists depending on the country to follow evidence-based prescribing. It was very interesting to hear students' experiences from different parts of the world where different prescribing rules apply. It is a very rewarding process but faces its own challenges.

Challenges

Data released in March 2023 by UCAS predicted that by 2030 we could see 30% more higher education applicants compared to 2022[8]. Biomedical science programmes are already very popular and demand is expected to grow. Classes often consist of large cohorts with a variety of learning experiences, especially at level four. Although students do want to be taught by experts, it is difficult to make sure that all students have equal opportunities to learn. It has previously been reported by many educationalists that large class sizes promote passive learning. However, with a growing number of students in Higher

Education, we are forced to identify a way to teach large classes without compromising intellectual engagement. In this case students enjoy analysing the three-D images of the biofilms and discover what is really like to be part of a biofilms using their own three-D glasses provided to them. This activity promotes engagement and a 'team chat' with their peers.

Embedding research in undergraduate learning, especially at level four, requires a conscious effort as it presents delivery constraints. The students need to develop a basic understanding of microbiology before they are exposed to the 'real' world. Therefore, the session is timetabled towards the end of the academic year, where (hopefully) most of the students are on a similar educational level.

Another challenge here is constantly updating/using technology. Technology insecurity can have an impact on lecturers' stress and anxiety[9]. Technology does have a didactic use but it can also affect academic staff, especially with the lack of technical resources. For example, when the laptop connected to the plate reader broke down, we discovered that our IT Department does not support it. Technology can come with a range of implications as well, including budget limitations. There is a constant pressure of exploring new research funding mechanisms and attracting internal and external income. This is a highly competitive process that often comes hand in hand with disappointment. There aren't many opportunities, or at least not as many as pre-Brexit. Also, money coming from industry very often comes with confidential agreements, which restricts research publication for any purpose. This leads to the following question: Should teaching be driving research funding allocation?

Acquiring, analysing and questioning knowledge is a key skill for a biomedical scientist. There is a diverse range of learning techniques but perhaps teaching students how to learn should be included in the traditional or research-integrated curricula[10].

Conclusion

Research-integrated teaching in biomedical science is an approach that deeply enriches the educational experience. It harmoniously bridges the gap between theoretical knowledge and the rapidly evolving landscape of biomedical research. By embedding the latest scientific advancements and methodologies directly into the curriculum, this approach ensures that students are not only well-informed but also actively engaged in the learning process. This method of teaching transforms students from passive learners into active participants, cultivating essential skills such as critical thinking, problem-solving, and innovative thinking. These skills are vital in a field that is characterised by swift advancements and complex challenges, such as those seen in genomics, cancer immunotherapy, and stem-cell technology. The integration of research into teaching also enables students to appreciate the dynamic and often debated nature of science, fostering a deeper understanding and a more nuanced perspective of the biomedical field.

Research-integrated teaching, however, comes with its own set of challenges, including ensuring the accessibility of complex research concepts to all students and creating assessments that accurately reflect this integrated approach. Overcoming these challenges requires thoughtful curriculum design, a collaborative effort among teaching staff, and a commitment to continual adaptation and improvement.

Ultimately, research-integrated teaching is not just beneficial but vital. It equips students with a robust and relevant education, preparing them to become the next generation of scientists who are capable of contributing to and advancing the field. By closely aligning academic learning with the forefront of scientific research, this approach prepares students not only for academic achievement but also for a successful and impactful career in biomedical science.

References

1. Nogrady B Rearranging the Building Blocks of Life. *Nature*. Published online 2019. Accessed February 1, 2023. https://www.nature.com/articles/d41586-019-01438-6.pdf

2. Burgum S, Stoakes G. What Does Research Informed Teaching Look Like. *The Higher Education Academy/University alliance*. Published online 2016. (Accessed: 20 August 2018). http://bit.ly/2h2JLke

3. Healey M Linking Research and Teaching: Exploring Disciplinary Spaces and the Role of Inquiry-Based Learning. Published online 2005. Accessed July 3, 2023. https://www.semanticscholar.org/paper/6274989392ec7f61bf0dc68e2719bd2789cd619b

4. Boyer EL. The Scholarship of Teaching From: Scholarship Reconsidered: Priorities of the Professoriate. *Coll Teach*. 1991;39(1):11–13.

5. Morris L Integrating Biomedical Engineering Research with Undergraduate Teaching – A Research-Teaching Nexus Approach. *Int J Cross-discip Subj Educ*. 2022;13(2):4692–4697.

6. Wainwright J, Hobbs G, Nakouti I. Persister Cells: Formation, Resuscitation and Combative Therapies. *Arch Microbiol*. 2021;203(10):5899–5906.

7. Hernández-Jiménez E, Del Campo R, Toledano V, et al. Biofilm vs. Planktonic Bacterial Mode of Growth: Which Do Human Macrophages Prefer? *Biochem Biophys Res Commun*. 2013;441(4):947–952.

8. UCAS. UCAS Kickstarts National Debate on Access to UK Higher Education as Competition Grows. *UCAS*. Published 27 March 2023. Accessed July 3, 2023. https://www.ucas.com/corporate/news-and-key-documents/news/ucas-kickstarts-national-debate-access-uk-higher-education-competition-grows

9. Fernández-Batanero JM, Román-Graván P, Reyes-Rebollo MM, Montenegro-Rueda M. Impact of Educational Technology on Teacher Stress and Anxiety: A Literature Review. *Int J Environ Res Public Health*. 2021;18(2). doi:10.3390/ijerph18020548

10. Franz A et al. How do medical students learn conceptual knowledge? High-, moderate- and low-utility learning techniques and perceived learning difficulties. *BMC Med Educ*. 2022;22(1):250.

4 Distributed learning

David I Lewis and Donna Johnson

What is distributed learning?

Distributed learning is a multimodal educational model that offers a nuanced blend of learning avenues and methodologies in order to cater to diverse learning preferences and schedules[1]. It includes both asynchronous and synchronous activities, enabling learners to engage in real-time interactions as well as self-paced learning. Asynchronous activities may include recorded lectures, readings, or discussion boards that students can access at any time, while synchronous activities involve real-time sessions such as webinars or live discussions.

The content in a distributed learning system is provided through a variety of channels and formats and these may include digital platforms like e-books or online articles, face-to-face classroom settings, as well as Virtual Learning Environments (VLEs), which offer a comprehensive digital space for educational interactions. These delivery mechanisms ensure that learners have the flexibility to engage with material in a way that suits them best. Distributed learning also accommodates both independent and collaborative forms of education. While some learners thrive in solo environments where they can delve deeply into topics, others benefit from team-based or social learning contexts where ideas can be exchanged and critiqued. In essence, this model encourages a harmonious blend of individual and collective learning experiences.

Importantly, distributed learning places a premium on learner autonomy, allowing individuals to participate according to their own schedules and at a pace that they find comfortable. This sense of ownership not only enhances their engagement but also instils a greater sense of responsibility for their educational journey. Students are thus empowered to tailor their learning experiences to their unique needs and aspirations, leading to more meaningful and enduring educational outcomes.

Creating inspirational student experiences

The goal of Higher Education is to develop Change Makers; graduates equipped with the experiences and competencies (knowledge, skills, and behaviours) to make a difference, able to contribute solutions to the many

DOI: 10.4324/9781003383994-7

complex problems facing the world. With increasing numbers of graduates going onto careers outside of their discipline, the development of these graduate core competencies is becoming more important than the acquisition of disciplinary-specific knowledge.

The UK secondary education system is designed to teach to the test, with learners assessed, through micro-assessments, on their ability to recall knowledge rather than their understanding of or ability to apply this knowledge. However, graduate employers require employees who have the competencies to discover, apply, and create new knowledge and understanding. It is therefore incumbent on university educators to bridge this gap by providing inspirational educational experiences, with appropriate scaffolding and support, a spiral curriculum that progressively develops the competencies and higher levels of learning required of graduates by employers.

Learner expectations have also changed[2]. They expect high-quality educational experiences which fully prepare them for the workplace and the diversity of careers they go onto, delivered in a manner and time which addresses their individual needs[3]. Increasing numbers of learners are undertaking part-time employment to support their studies or having caring or other responsibilities and therefore the traditional on-campus 9–5 curriculum is no longer fit for purpose.

Distributed learning plays a significant role in creating inspirational student experiences by offering a wide range of educational opportunities[3]. One of the most impactful aspects is the autonomy it offers learners. By allowing students to select their own pace, timing, and even the method of instruction, distributed learning fosters a sense of empowerment and ownership. This autonomy can serve as a powerful motivator, inspiring students to fully invest in their educational journey[4].

Distributed learning can also accommodate a wide array of learning styles and preferences – whether a student is more comfortable with independent study or thrives in a collaborative setting, the multimodal nature of this approach has something for everyone. This flexibility can ignite a passion for learning, as students find their individual needs met and their unique learning styles catered to[5].

The blend of various learning activities and formats in distributed learning enables us to provide authentic learning experiences, as they often mirror real-world scenarios. This practical application can imbue the learning experience with a sense of purpose and relevance, making it more meaningful and inspiring for students. The real-world applicability of the skills and knowledge gained can serve as a strong motivational factor, driving students to engage more deeply with the material[6].

Finally, the social components of distributed learning, such as peer discussions and group projects, create opportunities for interaction and collaboration. These social elements not only enrich the learning experience but also add an emotional layer that can be deeply inspiring. The chance to exchange ideas, receive feedback, and work collectively towards a common goal can stimulate intellectual curiosity and foster a sense of community, all factors that contribute to an engaging learning environment.

Distributed learning approaches

What do our learners think?

The switch to the use of online learning was rapid due to the pandemic. While lockdown was in place, online teaching was the only way we could continue to provide materials and support, but a large volume of online materials has remained in place even after a full return to campus. Feedback[7] has suggested that students were happy with the amount and quality of learning materials provided in lockdown, but what about now? Are they still as happy with working, at least partly, online?

Canvassing of student opinions of learning during and after the pandemic highlighted several positive aspects of online learning (flexibility and accessibility for example) but also a decrease in motivation and focus, particularly in first-year or younger students[7]. Online learning is also considered to provide fewer and lower-quality opportunities for interaction with peers and lecturers, and students still value the social aspects of being on campus[8]. With these outcomes, it seems reasonable that a distributed approach would be the best of both worlds, and this is reflected in student comments and results of larger-scale surveys, such as that carried out by the Joint Information Systems Committee (JISC)[9], where 71% of respondents agreed that the use of technology allowed them to make good progress with their learning.

However, it has not been a completely positive response from students, some just prefer in-person sessions, felt that recorded lectures contained too much information or were too fast-paced. Other students felt there was a disconnect between the online materials and in-person sessions supporting them. While many of these negative aspects highlighted by students come down to differences in personal preferences in their learning, they do highlight that one size doesn't fit all and that is something we need to take into consideration when we design the online parts of our teaching materials.

Challenges of using distributed approaches

There are a range of challenges associated with implementing distributed approaches. We can consider these in three categories:

- Institutional-based challenges
- Staff-based challenges
- Student-based challenges

Institutional-based challenges

Higher education institutes have increasingly moved towards distributed approaches as there is a continual requirement to develop teaching practices to fit better with student needs and desires and to make use of newer technologies. There was a complete switch to online teaching during the pandemic but many courses have chosen not to return back to running exactly the way they did before, instead keeping a more distributed approach. Such approaches have a number of benefits for an institution. They can be a way of managing increasing student numbers, make up for disparities in teaching room availability, and can help to decrease costs in some areas, however, there remain a number of challenges. Perhaps unsurprisingly, the main area of contention has been an institutional desire to keep a higher level of online provision, particularly for exams. This can be contrary to guidelines from accrediting bodies who feel that in person exams are a more robust mode of assessment than online exams. Accrediting bodies have supported the continuation of online assessments where there are pedagogical reasons for doing so and questions are designed to robustly assess ILOs without being easily Googleable/susceptible to breaches in academic integrity so providing assessments that tick all the boxes for all involved will remain a challenge.

In the UK, the availability of relevant technology at an institutional level is not generally an issue. We have suitable access to VLEs such as Blackboard or Moodle which have a range of tools built in that fit the bill. Where it becomes more difficult is where the infrastructure is not as built-in and for more practical-based subjects. For practical-based subjects, there are tools such as lab simulations available, but these, while useful, are often costly and pitched at an introductory level. There is widespread agreement about the benefit of actually doing the practical sessions in a lab so it's likely that distributed learning remains within the preparatory or reflective part of a lab activity.

Staff-based challenges

There has always been a mix of staff between those willing to try out new teaching technologies and those who prefer more traditional methods or just don't like online teaching. While the research on staff perceptions of distributed learning is extremely limited, a recent study by Anthony (2022)[10] suggests that social factors and interactions with colleagues can influence opinions and uptake – if colleagues use these approaches then others are more likely to consider also using it. Uptake is likely driven by intrinsic feelings about what distributed learning is as well – if staff like the idea of it then they're more likely to use it. This is combined with the perceptions of how complex it would be to use and the added value staff consider it to have[10].

Underpinning this is the general feeling towards and comfort with technology. Not all staff are sufficiently computer literate to have an easy transition into distributed learning. This was emphasised with the switch to online teaching during the pandemic[11]. While in general, students were happy with the level of online provision, there were reported margins between what was provided between modules and this was at least in part, down to the opinions and abilities of the staff involved[12]. There were teething problems as expected, particularly centred around availability/reliability of technology and connectivity and it was a steep learning curve when trying to learn to use the tools. Regardless of whether this is a case of can't rather than won't, the perception of students was that staff weren't bothered to make the effort to adapt nor to develop their skills for teaching online[13].

One thing we should be aware of is that our assumptions about the digital literacy of our students can be incorrect. We are mostly teaching students who have grown up in a more technological era than many of us and so the tendency can be to assume that students come to university fully equipped with the digital skills needed to succeed – that they are 'digital natives'. However, the concept of the 'digital native' has recently been debunked; the exposure to digital technologies, even from a very young age, does not equate to digital literacy[14]. If we continue to carry the assumption that it does, not only does this discount those mature students who grew up prior to this but also ignores the fact that students come from a wide variety of backgrounds, and many may be less able or less interested when it comes to use of technology, and even if they are regularly using social media, these skills don't necessarily translate to academic digital skills. Academic skills departments offer support for a wide range of digital topics and these continue to be widely accessed, even those that may be considered as fundamental knowledge[15]. This means that when we develop our teaching materials for distributed provision, we must ensure that there are clear instructions for their use and that we make them as accessible as possible.

Learner-based challenges

A particularly important learner challenge is digital poverty. A consequence of the increased provision of online materials and the continuation of a hybrid approach has highlighted issues with access and engagement for students facing socio-economic challenges, and these compound issues students may have already been facing if they have to work or have caring responsibilities or unsettled home lives[16]. Research published by the Office for Students suggests that over half of students have issues with slow or unreliable internet connections, 18% are impacted by having no access to the internet and 18% by having no access to a laptop, computer or tablet. Online learning also needs a suitable space but this has been an issue too, with nearly three-quarters of students reporting a problem here[17]. While there has been governmental support for colleges and schools[18], there has been nothing similar for higher education. Many universities have instituted digital hardship funds that have bridged some of the gaps and have a good level of on-campus computer and internet provision, but we must always be aware of issues with digital access when designing our distributed sessions.

Issues around access also feed into potential issues with balancing activities with the time they take. The intricacies surrounding digital access and time management in educational settings are far more nuanced than they might initially appear. On the surface, having good digital access – reliable internet connectivity and appropriate hardware – might seem like a solution to many of the challenges associated with distributed learning. However, this is only one part of a much larger equation. Even students who have robust internet connectivity may encounter difficulties when balancing the time needed to complete various activities. One reason for this is that having good digital access doesn't automatically equate to high digital literacy. Students may be familiar with browsing social media or using basic applications, but navigating an academic platform or using specialised software can be a different challenge altogether. For example, tasks that involve data analysis using specific software can be time-consuming for students unfamiliar with the interface, irrespective of how easily accessible the software is.

The quality of digital access is another factor that can impact time management. Internet speeds that are sufficient for basic activities like emailing or web browsing may be inadequate for more data-intensive tasks like streaming video lectures or participating in real-time collaborative projects. In such cases, students may find themselves spending a disproportionate amount of time waiting for videos to buffer or files to download, which can disrupt their schedule and impede their ability to manage their time effectively.

The flexibility that is often touted as an advantage of distributed learning can paradoxically become a hurdle when it comes to time management. Asynchronous learning environments, where students are free to access materials and complete tasks at their convenience, require strong self-discipline and time-management skills[19]. The absence of a fixed schedule can lead to procrastination, where students may delay tasks until they accumulate into an unmanageable workload. The asynchronous nature of many distributed learning courses can contribute to a misperception regarding the time needed for each task as well. An activity might seem simple when a student first encounters it on a learning platform, leading to the assumption that it will be quick to complete. However, once the student delves into the activity, it may turn out to be more complex and time-consuming than initially thought. This misjudgement can result in last-minute rushes and heightened stress levels as deadlines loom.

The design of the course itself can also contribute to these challenges. Educators who are new to distributed learning models may not accurately gauge the time commitment required for certain online tasks. For example, an instructor might assume that reading a 20-page journal article and completing an associated quiz would take a set amount of time, not considering the additional time students may need to decipher complex academic language or troubleshoot technical issues.

From a staff perspective probably the most frustrating student challenge is the often-low level of engagement with online materials and in online sessions. We spend a great deal of time and effort producing our materials only to see VLE reports suggesting that these are accessed only minimally if they are accessed at all. This lack of engagement is not only an issue of wasted resources; it has deeper ramifications for the learning process. When learners do not actively engage with the online materials, they miss out on essential components of the curriculum. This can result in a fragmented understanding of a topic, making it harder for them to grasp more complex, interrelated concepts they may cover later in the course. This lack of engagement often correlates with poor performance in assessments, creating a feedback loop of disengagement and academic struggle[20].

Several factors may contribute to the lack of engagement[21]. First, the impersonal nature of online learning environments can make learners feel disconnected, thereby reducing their motivation to engage with the materials. Second, the sheer volume of resources, which can be coupled with poor navigational structure in the VLE, can overwhelm learners, leading to overload. Finally, the absence of immediate accountability – unlike in a traditional classroom where a teacher might notice a student's lack of participation – can result in procrastination.

As educators, the challenge lies in developing strategies that result in greater engagement in the distributed learning arena. Some potential solutions include the gamification of learning materials[22], incorporating real-time analytics to provide immediate feedback, and using active learning strategies like flipped classrooms[23] to make online sessions more interactive. We also need to consider the emotional and psychological aspects of online learning, offering avenues for social interaction and emotional support[24].

Solutions and recommendations

Addressing the digital divide is an important step towards achieving equitable access to distributed learning. Institutions can provide devices for students to borrow and offer on-campus computer access but providing access to technology alone is not sufficient; students also need support in developing digital literacy skills to effectively navigate and use distributed learning environments. Online tutorials addressing digital skills have been shown to be effective[25], with many learners reporting enjoyment and ease of use, however, these have the same issues as distributed learning in general, with connectivity and hardware access potential issues. Gamification and peer–peer learning associated with digital literacy have also proven effective[26]. A further beneficial activity is integrating the development of digital literacy within the curriculum[27]. As well as developing necessary skills, learners have additional context for their importance, which in turn will promote engagement[6].

Staff may also benefit from access to this type of training opportunity – supporting staff development in the area of distributed learning is crucial for the success of distributed[28] learning initiatives. Increasing staff skills in this arena will increase confidence and perhaps enthusiasm about distributed learning technologies and this can in turn promote the development of new pedagogical practices that enhance student learning outcomes[28].

When it comes to fostering student engagement in a distributed learning environment, several strategies come to the fore. The integration of gamification elements into online activities, for example, has been shown to significantly boost student participation[29]. But engagement is not solely about individual interaction with the course material; it's also about building a community. Peer-to-peer interactions, facilitated through online discussion boards and collaborative projects, have been shown to enhance the sense of community, thereby increasing overall student engagement[30].

The provision of real-time feedback in online quizzes and assignments is also an important consideration in the context of distributed learning, and its impact on student satisfaction and engagement is supported by a wealth of evidence[31-33]. Real-time feedback acts as a form of validation for students, confirming whether their understanding of the material is accurate. This immediate gratification can be a powerful motivator, encouraging students to engage more deeply with the course content. It essentially creates a responsive learning environment where students are not just passive recipients of knowledge but active participants in a dynamic educational process. It also provides an opportunity for timely course correction. If a student is struggling with a particular concept, real-time feedback can alert both the learner and the educator to this issue before it becomes a significant obstacle to further learning. This allows for targeted interventions, such as additional resources or personalised instruction, to be implemented without delay. Real-time feedback can facilitate self-regulated learning as well, a key skill in any educational setting but particularly vital in distributed learning environments where students often study independently. By receiving real-time feedback, students can assess their own strengths and weaknesses in real time, adjusting their study strategies accordingly. This fosters a sense of autonomy and ownership over a learner's own educational journey, qualities that are strongly correlated with higher levels of engagement[34].

Adapting assessment methods to suit the unique characteristics of distributed learning environments is another area where we can support learners[35]. The incorporation of frequent formative assessments allows educators to gauge student understanding in real time, offering the flexibility to adapt teaching methods as the course progresses[32]. The use of diverse assessment methods, such as online quizzes, reflective journals, and group projects, can cater to a variety of learning styles. This not only accommodates different student preferences but also fosters the development of a broader skill set, including critical thinking and real-world application of knowledge[36].

Where possible it is beneficial to provide pre-recorded materials available for download. The availability of pre-recorded materials in easily digestible formats, such as podcasts and short screencasts, offers students the flexibility to engage with course content at their own pace. These materials, which should also be accessible via mobile devices, provide an additional layer of convenience, making it easier for students to integrate learning into their daily lives. This approach aligns well with evidence suggesting that multimodal and flexible learning pathways can significantly enhance the educational experience[37].

Case studies: Distributed learning in practice

Case study 1: Core concepts and their application in active learning workshops

DI Lewis and C Haigh
University of Leeds, UK

Scientific knowledge is increasing exponentially. Educators have historically dealt with this by increasing the content of the curriculum, in turn creating curriculum overload. Recognising this, PSRBs and Accrediting Bodies are increasingly moving away from defined curricula to an Intended Learning Outcomes (ILO) approach, leaving educators to decide which content or examples to include in their programmes to meet these broad ILOs. Whilst this may address the content overload issue, studies initially in physics undergraduate education and subsequently in biology education have shown that even the best prepared fourth-year students majoring in physics in elite US institutions were unable to apply key concepts in their discipline[38]. They had not developed effective conceptual frameworks required for human learning, and to be able to apply knowledge. To address this deficit, STEM educators are increasingly moving from content-driven to concept-driven programmes[39-43].

A core concept is defined as an indispensable idea that is key to both the understanding and execution within a particular field; attaining expertise in this aspect confers lasting comprehension and the aptitude to confront issues in that domain[44].

Core concepts (1–2 per podcast) are delivered in short (15 minute maximum) podcasts and made available to learners on the VLE at the beginning of each week. Concepts are illustrated using examples taken from the content of previous curricula and may be introduced at one level and developed in further levels, remain solely in one level, or be introduced in later levels of a programme. It is critical that where a concept forms part of an educational activity, it is identified in both the ILOs and during delivery, with links also made back to previous educational activities that included the concept. Learners can then assess their emerging knowledge and understanding through formative multiple-choice questions.

Critical to understanding a concept is the ability to apply it across different systems or topics, a competency that requires practice and appropriate scaffolding and support to develop. This is best developed through social or collaborative learning where team members help and support each other to create new knowledge and understanding. Individuals optimally acquire knowledge when they are proactive rather than passive, focused rather than diverted, and when the subject matter is coherent as opposed to fragmented. Additionally, the learning experience is most effective in a socially interactive setting that is based on iterative processes rather than simple repetition, all while maintaining an element of enjoyment[45].

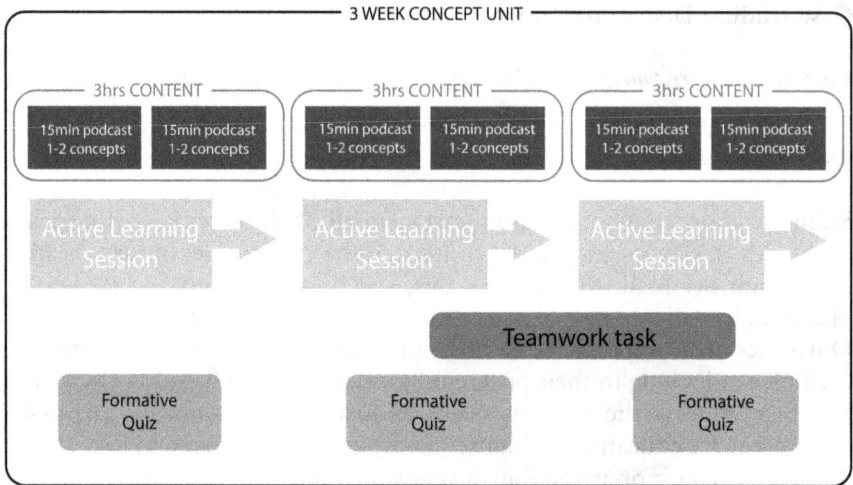

Figure 4.1 A structured educational framework for a three-week concept unit.

Teams of learners (4–6 per team) apply the concept(s) in in-person active learning plenary workshops to create solutions for example, to problem-solving exercises or case studies relevant to their discipline, sharing their solutions with the wider cohort (Figure 4.1). Individual activities encompass multiple concepts and topics enabling integration and application of learning. It is recommended that there be four hours of asynchronous content per two-hour workshop.

Case study 2: Experimental design-focused mini-projects

DI Lewis, D Donnelly and J Lippiat
University of Leeds, UK

In the biosciences, the development of experimental and technical skills is normally realised by learner participation in individual laboratory or fieldwork sessions or activities. These short sessions do not engage students, they often fail to see the link to other elements of their programme, and, recipe-driven, they do not provide the opportunity for learners to develop key research skills, for example, experimental design, or the formulation and testing of hypotheses.

These issues can be addressed through team-based pre-practical session activities where learning occurs before rather than during or after the experimental activity, and switching from individual practical experiences to experimental design-focused mini-projects.

In this social constructivism[46-48] model, teams of learners are provided with a problem or task, for example identifying, through *in-vitro* or *in-silico* approaches, an unknown pharmacological agent. The team then develops their research question and hypothesis, and gathers information from instructional techniques podcasts and other information sources to create their experimental plan which they submit (to other teams and the educational lead) for feedback and approval. They modify their plan, if required, based on this feedback and then test their hypothesis using *in-silico* and *in-vitro* approaches (e.g. simulations, existing datasets, data mining, laboratory sessions). Following this battery of experimental approaches, if they haven't identified their unknown pharmacological agent, they could reformulate their hypothesis and repeat the process until they create a solution. Each teams' challenges and their solutions are shared in a plenary wrap-up workshop.

This approach provides an inspirational and engaging educational experience that develops key competencies beyond experimental and technical skills and is preparation for their final year or Honours capstone project and future careers. It enables the introduction of authentic and attribute-focused assessments, for example, experimental plans with budgets and milestones, academic papers or Briefing Notes for Regulators rather than the traditional laboratory or fieldwork report. It is also resource-light, freeing up laboratory, educator and technical support staff time.

Case study 3: Team-based social justice or UN sustainable development goal challenges using design thinking approaches

A Holmes
University of Leeds, UK

A Drovandi
University of Manchester, UK

DI Lewis
University of Leeds, UK

Employers are increasingly requiring graduates that are socially responsible, and globally culturally aware. The revised QAA Benchmarks[49] require the inclusion of Education for Sustainable Development and Equity, Diversity and Inclusion educational experiences. Traditional undergraduate skills modules or courses rarely develop these social justice competencies.

Design Thinking[50] is a team-based approach used in industry to create innovative and creative solutions to problems or challenges. It is an inclusive approach that emphasises to stakeholders that everybody's opinion is equally valued and respected and results in solutions that fully address all stakeholders' needs.

Teams (4–6) of learners are provided with a Glocal (global at a local, community level, e.g. Healthy ageing) or UN Sustainable Development Goal[51] (UN SDG, e.g. a disease or disorder prevalent or a significant challenge in an identified resource-constrained Global South country). They identify stakeholders, empathising with them and identifying the challenges they face. They then discover and evaluate information to create evidence-informed solutions for each stakeholder community. Solutions are tested and refined, potentially requiring going back to the challenges phase, before SMART[52] recommendations are created.

The assessment is the team creation of a reflective e-portfolio and an individual portfolio showcasing their contributions to the team's output, and the development of their individual competencies.

This activity requires appropriate scaffolding and support. Each stage is supported by synchronous and asynchronous activities and resources that develop the key competencies required (e.g. project planning and organisation, information searching, critical thinking). They are provided with suggested stakeholder lists and information sources, plenary workshops to apply these competencies, and timetabled in-person team-working sessions (all teams present in a large flat seminar space), facilitated by a mentor, for teams to work on their project.

Case study 4: Team-based education for sustainable development, trans-national capstone experiences

DI Lewis
University of Leeds, UK

HO Kwanashie, SU Adamu, GO Anetor
National Open University of Nigeria, Nigeria

H Campbell, S Chakrabarty
University of Leeds, UK

EM Joseph-Shehu
National Open University of Nigeria, Nigeria

R Norman
University of Leeds, UK

GI Okoroiwu, O Saliu
National Open University of Nigeria, Nigeria

C Tweedy
University of Leeds, UK

F Uchendu
National Open University of Nigeria, Nigeria

To fully raise awareness of different cultures and communities, and to develop Global Graduates, requires immersion in a community-engaged transnational educational experience, collaborating, in equal partnership, with learners from a different culture and continent, for example Global North with Global South.

Grand Challenges capstones are where teams of learners from a Global South institution and a Global North Institution work collaboratively together to co-create an evidence-driven report, with recommendations, which offers frugal (affordable, capable of implementation in both countries) solutions to an identified UN SDG[51] or Global Grand Challenge[53] relevant to both countries.

Team members meet to introduce themselves, share their goals, ambitions and concerns for the project, and agree on the project timelines, milestones and digital communication tools they will use. They then are provided with a list of disciplinary relevant challenges to choose from. They use a Design Thinking[54] approach to identify stakeholders, empathise with them and identify their challenges, discover and evaluate information to create evidence-informed solutions and SMART[52] recommendations.

The use of the Design Thinking[50] approach means that team members from different Institutions do not have to start at the same time, a common occurrence within trans-national educational opportunities with differing dates for the academic year. If the members from one institution have started, when the second Institution joins, the team quickly return to the stakeholder identification stage. Previous work is not wasted, they just modify the stakeholder list (and all subsequent stages) in light of the joining members' expertise and lived experiences. This process actually broadens cultural awareness and understanding. Likewise, they do not have to end at the same time. Provided the team has completed the evidence-gathering and solution-creation stage, there is sufficient information for individual team members to create their own recommendations and written outputs.

Learners reflect regularly on their experiences, and on their learning about themselves and others, and apply this learning to the next stage of the Design Thinking[54] process. Critical to this learning and personal development is giving learners and teams ownership and responsibility for their experiences. Therefore, educators should act as mentors not supervisors, allowing learners to make mistakes, to reflect on them and learn from them.

Virtual mini-symposia at the empathy and solutions stages, where teams share their plans and outputs respectively with other teams for feedback and comments provides a supportive opportunity for formative feedback and progress checking.

The suggested output for this activity is a reflective e-portfolio where learners cannot only showcase their outputs but also the competencies they have developed, their reflections on their learning and experiences, and how they have applied these throughout the project. However, Institutional requirements may vary and therefore alternative assessment approaches are a business-style report, a dissertation or an academic paper. It is perfectly acceptable for different team members to choose different assessment tools, the one that they are most comfortable with and which best showcases their competencies to potential employers.

Conclusion

Distributed learning emerges as a transformative approach that adeptly addresses the needs of a diverse student population. This educational model, with its blend of asynchronous and synchronous methods, presents a solution that caters to various learning preferences and schedules, offering a more inclusive and accessible learning environment. Central to its success is its emphasis on learner autonomy and customisation, empowering students and providing them with the agency to shape their educational experiences in ways that align with their personal needs and goals. It is especially pertinent in biomedical science education, bridging the gap between traditional academic instruction and the practical competencies required in the field. Distributed learning, therefore, not only imparts knowledge but also develops essential skills, preparing students for diverse and evolving career paths.

Implementing distributed learning is not without its challenges, which manifest at various levels – institutional, staff, and student. Institutions must navigate the integration of new teaching models and compliance with accreditation standards. Staff members are required to adapt to technological advancements and evolving teaching methodologies. Students, on the other hand, face challenges such as digital inequality and the need for effective self-management in an autonomous learning environment. To maximise the potential of distributed learning, it is important to address these challenges comprehensively. Enhancing digital access and literacy, facilitating staff development in distributed learning technologies, and promoting student engagement through interactive and responsive online elements are critical. Adapting assessment methods to align with the distinctive characteristics of distributed learning environments can further enhance its effectiveness as well.

Overall, distributed learning stands as a progressive and adaptable educational model, offering significant promise for the future of biomedical science education. Its capacity to meet a broad spectrum of learning needs and preferences positions it as a key component in the ongoing evolution of educational practices, promising to enhance the learning experience and outcomes for a wide range of learners.

References

1. Victor S, Hart S. Distributed learning: A flexible learning and development model. In: *E-Learn: World Conference on E-Learning in Corporate, Government, Healthcare, and Higher Education*. Association for the Advancement of Computing in Education (AACE); 2016:281–290.
2. Gorgodze S, Macharashvili L, Kamladze A. Learning for earning: Student expectations and perceptions of university. *Int Educ Stud*. 2019;13(1):42.
3. Lewis DI. Post-COVID education: eLearning and the new world of education. *Pharmacology Matters*. Published online 2020.
4. Marshik T, Ashton PT, Algina J. Teachers' and students' needs for autonomy, competence, and relatedness as predictors of students' achievement. *Soc Psychol Educ*. 2017;20(1):39–67.
5. Shuja A, Qureshi IA, Schaeffer DM, Zareen M. Effect of M-learning on students' academic performance mediated by facilitation discourse and flexibility. *Knowl Manag E-Learn*. 2019;11(2):158–200.
6. Erbaggio P, Gopalakrishnan S, Hobbs S, Liu H. Enhancing student engagement through online authentic materials. *IALLT J Lang Learn Technol*. 2012;42(2):27–51.

7. Stevanović A, Božić R, Radović S. Higher education students' experiences and opinion about distance learning during the Covid-19 pandemic. *J Comput Assist Learn.* 2021;37(6):1682–1693.
8. Sharma D, Sood AK, Darius PSH, Gundabattini E, Darius Gnanaraj S, Joseph JeyapaulA. A study on the online-offline and blended learning methods. *Journal of The Institution of Engineers (India): Series B.* 2022;103(4):1373–1382.
9. Knight S University students are happier with online learning post-pandemic. *Jisc.* Accessed September 25, 2023. https://beta.jisc.ac.uk/news/all/university-students-are-happier-with-online-learning-post-pandemic
10. Anthony Jnr. B An exploratory study on academic staff perception towards blended learning in higher education. *Educ Inf Technol.* 2022;27(3):3107–3133.
11. Almahasees Z, Mohsen K, Amin MO. Faculty's and students' perceptions of online learning during COVID-19. *Front Educ.* 2021;6. doi:10.3389/feduc.2021.638470
12. Nicklin LL, Wilsdon L, Chadwick D, et al. Accelerated HE digitalisation: Exploring staff and student experiences of the COVID-19 rapid online-learning transfer. *Educ Inf Technol (Dordr).* 2022;27(6):7653–7678.
13. Coman C, Ţîru LG, Meseşan-Schmitz L, Stanciu C, Bularca MC. Online teaching and learning in higher education during the coronavirus pandemic: Students' perspective. *Sustain Sci Pract Policy.* 2020;12(24):10367.
14. Reid L, Button D, Brommeyer M. Challenging the myth of the digital native: A narrative review. *Nurs Rep.* 2023;13(2):573–600.
15. Farrell LG. Challenging assumptions about IT skills in higher education. *JLDHE.* 2013;6. doi:10.47408/jldhe.v0i6.173
16. Butcher J, Curry G. Digital poverty as a barrier to access. *Widening Participation and Lifelong Learning.* 2022;24(2):180–194.
17. Office for Students. 'Digital poverty' risks leaving students behind. https://www.officeforstudents.org.uk/news-blog-and-events/press-and-media/digital-poverty-risks-leaving-students-behind/. Published 3 September 2020. Accessed April 10, 2021.
18. Get help with technology: conditions of internet access and device grants. *Gov.uk.* Published 29 October 2021. Accessed March 29, 2023. https://www.gov.uk/government/publications/get-help-with-technology-conditions-of-internet-access-and-device-grants
19. Muksin SNB, Makhsin MB. A level of student self-discipline in E-learning during pandemic covid-19. *Procedia Soc Sci Humanit.* 2021;1:278–283.
20. Atherton M, Shah M, Vazquez J, Griffiths Z, Jackson B, Burgess C. Using learning analytics to assess student engagement and academic outcomes in open access enabling programmes. *Open Learning: J Open, Dist e-Learning.* 2017;32(2):119–136.
21. Adeshola I, Agoyi M. Examining factors influencing e-learning engagement among university students during covid-19 pandemic: A mediating role of "learning persistence". *Interactive Learning Environments.* Published online 2022:1–28.
22. Smiderle R, Rigo SJ, Marques LB, Peçanha de Miranda Coelho JA, Jaques PA. The impact of gamification on students' learning, engagement and behavior based on their personality traits. *Smart Learn Environ.* 2020;7(1). doi:10.1186/s40561-019-0098-x
23. Smallhorn M The flipped classroom: A learning model to increase student engagement not academic achievement. *Stud Success.* 2017;8(2):43–53.
24. Mheidly N, Fares MY, Fares J. Coping with stress and burnout associated with telecommunication and online learning. *Front Public Health.* 2020;8:574969.
25. McGuinness C, Fulton C. Digital literacy in higher education: A case study of student engagement with e-tutorials using blended learning. *J Inf Technol Educ: Innov Pract.* 2019;18:1–28.

26. Kulju P, Mäkinen M. Phonological strategies and peer scaffolding in digital literacy game-playing sessions in a Finnish pre-primary class. *J Early Child Lit.* 2021;21(3): 338–360.

27. Hinrichsen J, Coombs A. The five resources of critical digital literacy: A framework for curriculum integration. *Res Learn Technol.* 2013;21. doi:10.3402/rlt.v21.21334

28. Romero-Hall E, Jaramillo CherrezN. Teaching in times of disruption: Faculty digital literacy in higher education during the COVID-19 pandemic. *Innov Educ Teach Int.* 2023;60(2):152–162.

29. Bouchrika I, Harrati N, Wanick V, Wills G. Exploring the impact of gamification on student engagement and involvement with e-learning systems. *Interact Learn Environ.* 2021;29(8):1244–1257.

30. McFarlane R, Spes-Skrbis M, Taib A. Let's Chat-A fresh take on the invaluable role of peer-to-peer conversation in student engagement, participation and inclusion. *Student success.* Published online 2017. https://search.informit.org/doi/abs/10. 3316/informit.593553318056413

31. Suraworachet W, Zhou Q, Cukurova M. Impact of combining human and analytics feedback on students' engagement with, and performance in, reflective writing tasks. *Int J Educ Technol High.* 2023;20(1):1–24.

32. Shute VJ. Focus on formative feedback. *Rev Educ Res.* 2008;78(1):153–189.

33. Asiri YA, Millard DE, Weal MJ. Assessing the impact of engagement and real-time feedback in a mobile behavior change intervention for supporting critical thinking in engineering research projects. *IEEE Trans Learn Technol.* 2021;14(4). https:// ieeexplore.ieee.org/document/9513591

34. Alley KM. Fostering middle school students' autonomy to support motivation and engagement. *Middle Sch J.* 2019;50(3):5–14.

35. Fjørtoft H Multimodal digital classroom assessments. *Comput Educ.* 2020;152:103892.

36. Wekerle C, Daumiller M, Kollar I. Using digital technology to promote higher education learning: The importance of different learning activities and their relations to learning outcomes. *J Res Technol Educ.* 2022;54(1):1–17.

37. Qushem UB, Christopoulos A, Oyelere SS, Ogata H, Laakso MJ. Multimodal technologies in precision education: Providing new opportunities or adding more challenges? *Educ Sci.* 2021;11(7):338.

38. Hestenes D Toward a modeling theory of physics instruction. *Am J Phys.* 1987;55(5):440–454.

39. Lynn Erickson H, Lanning LA. *Transitioning to Concept-Based Curriculum and Instruction: How to Bring Content and Process Together.* Corwin Press; 2013.

40. Baron KA. Changing to concept-based curricula: The process for nurse educators. *Open Nurs J.* 2017;11:277.

41. Merkel S, ASM task force on curriculum guidelines for undergraduate microbiology. The development of curricular guidelines for introductory microbiology that focus on understanding. *J Microbiol Biol Educ.* 2012;13(1):32–38.

42. Tansey JT, Baird T Jr, Cox MM, et al. Foundational concepts and underlying theories for majors in 'biochemistry and molecular biology'. *Biochem Mol Biol Educ.* 2013;41(5):289–296.

43. White PJ, Guilding C, Angelo T, et al. Identifying the core concepts of pharmacology education: A global initiative. *Br J Pharmacol.* 2023;180(9):1197–1209.

44. McFarland JL, Michael JA. Reflections on core concepts for undergraduate physiology programs. *Adv Physiol Educ.* 2020;44(4):626–631.

45. Zosh JM, Hirsh-Pasek K, Hopkins EJ, et al. Accessing the inaccessible: Redefining play as a spectrum. *Front Psychol.* 2018;9:1124.
46. Salmons J E-social constructivism and collaborative E-learning. In: Khosrow-Pour, Mehdi, Kamel, Sherif, Jerzy Kisielnicki, In Lee, Siau, Keng, Gupta, Amar, van Slyke, Craig, Wang, John, Weerakkody, Vishanth, Clarke, Steve, Jennex, Murray E., Becker, Annie, Anttiroiko, Ari-Veikko (Eds). *Instructional Design: Concepts, Methodologies, Tools and Applications.* IGI Global; 2011:1730–1743.
47. Lewis DI. Repository of open access datasets and tools. Google Docs. Published 2020. Accessed October 17, 2023. https://docs.google.com/spreadsheets/d/1rOnsON3-JFbACrrEl8QoAKThkZmN-wLewnD5Egm2Apc/edit
48. Lewis DI. e-biopracticals. Google Docs. Published 2020. Accessed October 17, 2023. https://docs.google.com/spreadsheets/d/1eqkpRq_OXgLzmb3rcK32Pe kdCakcpmUq67hpOGrj3OI/edit
49. Qaa. UK quality code for higher education. Part A: Setting and maintaining academic standards. *The Frameworks for Higher Education Qualifications of UK Degree-Awarding Bodies.* Published online 2014.
50. Morgan T, Jaspersen LJ. *Design thinking for student projects.* SAGE Publications Ltd. Published 8 October 2023. Accessed October 13, 2023. https://uk.sagepub.com/en-gb/eur/design-thinking-for-student-projects/book276875
51. THE 17 GOALS. Accessed October 9, 2023. https://sdgs.un.org/goals
52. Leonard K The ultimate guide to S.M.A.R.T. goals. *Forbes Magazine.* Published online 4 May 2022. Accessed October 9, 2023. https://www.forbes.com/advisor/business/smart-goals/
53. Global Grand Challenges. Accessed October 9, 2023. https://gcgh.grandchallenges.org/
54. Razzouk R, Shute V. What is design thinking and why is it important? *Rev Educ Res.* 2012;82(3):330–348.

5 Teaching practical skills to undergraduate biomedical science students

Ian Hurley, Wayne Roberts and Donna Johnson

The importance of practical skills

The development of practical skills in biomedical science degrees is vital. A majority of graduates will pursue lab-based or similar careers, and these require a strong skillset in fundamental lab techniques as well as the theoretical background. Practical sessions also promote the development of critical thinking, data analysis and communication, all key skills for employment[1]. However, the way we approach teaching these skills can have a significant impact on the learning outcomes of our students, and the more traditional lab-book-based approach can often leave students unengaged and dissatisfied. This is a disappointing outcome for both staff and students as the labs should be one of the most enjoyable components of a biomedical science degree.

However, the pedagogical approaches to imparting these skills can profoundly influence student learning outcomes. Traditional methods, such as lab-book-based instruction, can sometimes result in student disengagement and dissatisfaction, undermining what should be one of the most engaging aspects of a biomedical science degree. Getting the basics right is crucial. Fundamental skills like pipette usage, microscope operation, and spectrophotometry are not just foundational; they are also versatile, with applications across various scientific disciplines. This cross-applicability enhances employability and aligns with the Quality Assurance Agency for Higher Education (QAA) and Institute of Biomedical Science (IBMS) guidelines[2-4], which stress the importance of being conversant with contemporary laboratory methods for diagnosing and monitoring human health and disease.

Practical work, whether conducted in labs, or through *in silico* methods like modelling and data mining, serves multiple educational objectives. It not only reinforces the taught curriculum but also provides students with an understanding of the inherent variability in biological systems, along with the statistical methods to manage this variability. It also equips students with the competencies required in their chosen subject area, including the planning and execution of research projects, adherence to good laboratory practice, and awareness of health, safety, legal, and ethical considerations.

DOI: 10.4324/9781003383994-8

Considerations for teaching practical skills

Teaching practical skills in biomedical science poses several challenges as it is a multidisciplinary and rapidly evolving field. Biomedical science integrates various scientific disciplines, necessitating the coverage of a wide range of techniques, such as molecular biology, histology, and microscopy. This diverse knowledge base is essential for students to develop a comprehensive understanding of the subject. Ensuring that students have a strong foundation in these areas is vital, as inadequate fundamental skills can lead to difficulties at more advanced levels. To address this issue, we can employ strategies that promote active learning and develop critical thinking, such as problem-based learning, case studies, and inquiry-based approaches. We can also reinforce student understanding by providing additional resources, such as tutorials and preparatory materials[5]. Technology, such as virtual labs, online simulations, and digital microscopy, can further enhance the learning experience and facilitate the acquisition of practical skills. These tools can enable students to practice techniques and develop their skills in their own time and at their own pace, thus better preparing them for the lab-based sessions and more advanced skills[6].

When working in the lab, students must learn to handle potentially hazardous materials and equipment. In both the preparation and execution, ensuring safety is time-consuming and requires the support of additional staff in the lab sessions. To ensure safety and competence, we need to provide clear guidelines as well as comprehensive training. This can include hands-on demonstrations, instructional videos, or even online modules to reinforce proper practices. Ensuring students are being safe in the lab is not a one-and-done objective, we need to embed safety guidance within all of our lab materials and undergo regular monitoring of student progress to help identify areas where additional training may be needed.

Linking practical skills to other course content and the research project is essential to demonstrate their relevance and enhance knowledge retention. However, this can be challenging, as the practical components may seem disconnected from the theoretical aspects of the course. In order to try and avoid this issue we can design a practical curriculum that systematically builds upon previously learned material that is clearly signposted within both the practical and theoretical sessions.

Ensuring that the content is pitched at the right level for students and the course is vital to avoid overwhelming or under-challenging them and ensure they are developing a robust foundation. In a typical practical curriculum, skills progress from basic to more advanced as students advance through their course. This progression allows students to build on their foundational skills and gain greater independence in applying these skills to increasingly complex problems.

At level four, students might focus on acquiring basic skills such as pipetting, preparing solutions, using basic equipment (e.g., centrifuges, spectrophotometers), and following established protocols. The teaching approach may be more guided, with us providing step-by-step instructions and demonstrations. However, students can still be encouraged to engage in investigative activities, such as designing simple experiments, analysing data, and drawing conclusions based on their findings.

As students progress to level five, they may be introduced to more advanced techniques, such as gel electrophoresis, Polymerase Chain Reaction (PCR), cell culture, and histological staining. With a stronger foundation in basic skills, students can be given less guidance and more opportunities to explore the techniques independently or in small groups. They could be given trouble-shooting or optimisation experiments to develop critical thinking skills and be provided with more complex data for interpretation.

At level six, students will have developed a good foundation in the practical and theoretical aspects of their course, and we should be encouraging them to work with greater independence, particularly within their research projects. In addition to the research project, students will typically also be carrying out more advanced experiments in their subject-specific modules. If we can strengthen the links between these further at level six we can ensure that students develop the best mindset for seeking work after graduation.

If we combine the progressive development of skills with guided opportunities for reflection, we can further emphasise links between content and practical skills, ultimately enhancing students' learning experience and long-term retention. Reflective practice encourages students to think critically about their experiences and learning, leading to a deeper understanding and more effective learning[7].

The financial cost of including practical components in the curriculum can be considerable, as equipment, consumables, and facility maintenance can be expensive. We will be pushed to be mindful of budgetary constraints and so will need to seek creative ways to provide hands-on experiences for our students without compromising the quality of their education. There will be multiple approaches we can take to achieve this, such as integration of open education materials or lab simulations or we can explore the possibility of collaboration with other universities for resource sharing[6].

Organising and running lab sessions can be time-consuming for us and our students. To address this, we need to develop efficient workflows and protocols and adopt teaching strategies such as the flipped classroom, which allows students to learn theoretical concepts outside the classroom and dedicate class time to hands-on activities[8].

An especially challenging aspect of practical skills development within the curriculum is the assessment. Assessing practical skills often involves observation of our student's performance in the lab which is time-consuming and can be subjective. Staff may have different opinions on the quality of a student's work, making it difficult to ensure consistency and fairness in marking. To address this issue, we need to develop clear rubrics that outline specific criteria and performance standards for practical skills assessment. Assessing the diverse array of skills embedded in a biomedical science degree can be challenging as well, as it requires a comprehensive understanding of each technique and the ability to evaluate student performance across multiple domains. We can address this by including a range of assessment methods, such as exams, lab reports, and presentations, to enable us to evaluate different aspects of students' practical skills[9,10].

Teaching practical skills

Teaching practical skills effectively often requires a mixed approach, incorporating elements of constructivism and experiential/active learning. Constructivism emphasises the importance of students actively constructing knowledge through hands-on experiences and problem-solving[11], while experiential learning highlights the value of learning from direct experience and reflection[12].

Providing students with multiple opportunities to practice and refine their skills in different contexts will lead to more effective practical skills development. Multiple attempts for practical activities not only help students to learn from their mistakes but also enable them to build confidence in their abilities. These varied experiences also facilitate the transfer of skills from one context to another, which is an essential aspect of learning[13,14]. If we include similar lab activities in a range of contexts then students will be better able to see the relevance and applicability of the skills they are learning. This process helps them to more effectively connect theoretical knowledge with practical experiences, making it easier for them to understand the underlying principles and concepts. It also exposes them to different problem-solving strategies and encourages them to think critically and creatively about the tasks at hand. This exposure fosters the development of higher-order thinking skills, which are essential for success in both academic and professional settings[15].

Clear Intended Learning Objectives (ILOs) are essential for guiding the teaching process in the lab. ILOs will often emphasise the development of specific practical skills and/or data interpretation. They provide a comprehensive framework that helps our students understand what they are expected to learn and achieve in the lab, ensuring a more focused and efficient learning experience[16]. If we include them prominently in the lab teaching materials and go over them at the start of each lab session students will better understand the purpose and goals of the session, enabling them to focus their efforts on achieving the desired outcomes[17]. Incorporating ILOs into the lab teaching materials can also enhance their effectiveness as learning tools. When students document their work and reflect on their progress in relation to the ILOs, they can better identify areas for improvement and receive more targeted feedback from staff. This process of self-assessment and reflection is essential for developing students' metacognitive skills and fostering a growth mindset[18]. Clear ILOs will also provide a basis for communication between us and our students. By covering the ILOs during lab sessions, students can ask questions to clarify their understanding and receive immediate guidance. This ongoing dialogue can foster a collaborative learning environment, in which students feel supported and encouraged to take responsibility for their own learning[19].

ILOs are useful for us as well. We can use them to guide the design of lab activities and assessments and by doing so, ensure that the tasks and rubrics align clearly with them. This clarity creates a coherent and meaningful learning experience for our students and is crucial for promoting deep learning, as it encourages students to engage with the material in a way that promotes the development of the targeted skills and competencies[20].

The importance of lab books

A well-structured lab book is an indispensable tool for teaching practical skills. It serves multiple functions that go beyond being a repository for experimental data. Firstly, a lab book acts as a permanent record of all the experiments conducted in the lab. This function is crucial for both students and educators, as it allows for the tracking of work overtime, providing a detailed account of what was done, how it was done, and what the outcomes were. This documentation of work in a lab book extends to the realm of academic integrity and accountability as well. Should questions arise about the validity or replicability of an experiment, the lab book serves as an official record that can be consulted. In professional settings, maintaining a detailed lab book is often a regulatory requirement, making the practice of keeping one an essential skill that students should acquire during their education.

A well-organised lab book serves as a reflective tool for students. By regularly updating their lab books and reviewing past entries, students can engage in self-assessment, gauging their progress over the course of their studies. This reflective practice can be instrumental in identifying strengths and weaknesses, allowing students to focus on areas that require improvement. We can also use these lab books to provide targeted feedback, further aiding in student development. Lab books can also be a valuable learning resource in their own right. They can help students prepare for exams by serving as a study guide that includes not just theoretical knowledge, but also practical insights gained from hands-on experience.

Students won't necessarily know how to keep a comprehensive lab book so it's important for us to provide guidance on how to maintain one effectively. This could include dedicated sessions on lab book management, templates that guide students on what to include in each entry, along with periodic reviews to ensure that students are keeping up with best practices.

As students progress through their degree, the lab book should evolve to reflect their increasing knowledge and skills. At level four, lab books should focus on basic experimental techniques, safety procedures, and documentation practices. Students should be introduced to the importance of clear and accurate record-keeping and encouraged to document each step of the experimental process, including the materials used, the procedures followed, and the results obtained.

At level five, lab books should build on the skills learned at level four, with a greater emphasis on experimental design, data analysis, and critical thinking.

Students should be encouraged to develop their own research questions, design experiments to test these questions, and analyse and interpret the resulting data. Lab books should also include more detailed explanations of the theoretical concepts behind the experiments, helping students to connect the practical skills they are developing with the underlying scientific principles.

At level six, lab books should reflect the advanced knowledge and skills that students have acquired throughout their degree program. Lab books should focus on experimental design and execution, with a particular emphasis on developing independent research projects. Students should be encouraged to document their entire research process, including background reading, hypothesis development, experimental design, data collection, analysis, and interpretation. Lab books should also include detailed discussions of the broader implications of the research, including its relevance to current scientific debates and potential applications in industry or clinical practice.

The importance of preparation

Student preparation for learning lab skills is crucial, especially in complex fields like biomedical science where hands-on experience is vital for understanding the concepts and post-graduation employment.

The success of student preparation in learning practical skills is well-documented and has shown a clear positive impact on both academic achievement and real-world application abilities. A study by Stieff et al. (2018) assessed how preparatory activities influenced students' lab performance. They found that those students who engaged in preparatory work were better able to apply their theoretical knowledge during lab sessions. The preparatory activities facilitated familiarity with the contents of the lab, decreasing anxiety and increasing confidence, which in turn led to increased effectiveness in the lab. This then resulted in better quality work and improved student outcomes. They also highlighted the role of preparation in supporting students' lab skills and enabling them to translate theoretical knowledge into real-world scenarios. This not only boosted academic performance but also equipped students with a robust understanding of how to practically implement their knowledge, preparing them for employment[21].

A meta-analysis conducted by Hattie et al. (1996) further supported the significance of student preparation on academic achievement. They reported that students participating in preparatory activities showed a better overall performance compared to their non-preparatory classmates. The preparatory activities fostered a deeper understanding of the material and encouraged active learning. Preparation enabled students to organise their time more efficiently, more effectively understand the objectives of the lab session, and engage better with the material[22].

Integrating lab sessions with theoretical knowledge is a vital strategy for enhancing student preparation. If we can link a lab session to a specific taught session and then introduce the lab at the end of it, we can demonstrate the direct connection between the abstract concepts and their practical applications. This practice not only bridges the gap between theory and practice but also deepens students' understanding of the material. According to a study by Robertson (1997), students who saw a clear link between theory and practice showed improved comprehension and retention of course material[23].

Engaging students in quizzes or short activities prior to the lab is another effective strategy. Such activities will serve as both an assessment understanding of the theoretical material and a measure of their preparedness for the lab. They also help students identify areas they need to review before the lab and completion of the quizzes perform better in the subsequent lab session than those who did not[24].

Making a lab book available before the lab session is crucial. This allows students to read through the procedures and familiarise themselves with session content and objectives. If we also link the lab book to quizzes and other preparatory activities, then we can further reinforce students' understanding of the lab content. We should include the ILOs for the lab in the lab book. If we do this, they can guide students in their preparation. This also allows students to understand the purpose of the lab, what they will be learning, and what they will be expected to do. This can help them focus their preparation efforts on the most important aspects of the lab.

The use of multimedia resources, such as relevant videos and lab simulations, can also greatly enhance student preparation. These resources provide a visual representation of the lab procedures, which can make the abstract concepts more concrete and accessible. They can also help reduce students' anxiety about the lab by familiarising them with what they can expect when they get to the lab. Research has shown that the use of lab simulations before the lab session led to a better understanding of the lab procedures and performed better in the lab[25,26].

A key concern is the extent to which students engage with the preparatory activities we provide. If we include the preparatory activities as a component of the module mark this can be effective in motivating students to take the preparatory activities seriously. This strategy can increase students' engagement with these materials and improve their overall preparedness for the lab session.

Data analysis and interpretation

Data analysis and interpretation are fundamental skills that students need to master. The constraints of lab time make it even more critical to ensure that students are well-prepared before they set foot in the lab. This preparation should be comprehensive, extending beyond the basic orientation on lab equipment and procedures. Students should be trained in the methods and techniques of data analysis and interpretation, which are integral to the scientific process.

The importance of these skills is multi-faceted. In a clinical environment, the ability to interpret lab results accurately is not just an academic exercise; it has real-world implications, potentially affecting patient diagnoses and treatment plans. Similarly, in research settings, robust data analysis skills are essential for the credibility and impact of the study. A poorly analysed dataset can undermine the validity of research findings, regardless of how well the experiment was conducted.

Beyond these specific applications, data interpretation also serves to enhance critical thinking skills. It teaches students to scrutinise data, identify patterns or anomalies, and draw reasoned conclusions. These are transferable skills that are valuable not just in scientific research but also in various professional roles that students may take up after graduation.

There are many strategies we could use to enable students to better prepare for their data analysis task, from offering online tutorials that students can access before the lab sessions to providing interactive simulations that mimic real-world scenarios. Problem-solving exercises that require data interpretation can also be beneficial, as they allow students to apply theoretical knowledge in a practical context. These preparatory activities serve to maximise the use of the limited lab time, enabling students to focus on the more complex aspects of data analysis and interpretation rather than just the mechanics of data collection.

Case study – An outbreak of an antibiotic-resistant bacterial infection

The progressive development of lab skills is a fundamental aspect of biomedical science education and is critical for students' overall learning process. It mirrors the gradual acquisition of knowledge and skills in the theoretical aspects, where we establish fundamental knowledge and understanding and then move to more advanced concepts[27].

In the context of lab skills, students need to start with basic techniques at level four and then as students advance through their course, their lab skills are expected to grow in complexity. At intermediate levels, students will be exposed to more sophisticated experiments and use more specialised methods. During this phase, the emphasis shifts from simply carrying out the method to understanding when and why to use them, and how to interpret the results. This level of understanding is critical for developing problem-solving skills and the ability to think critically about experimental design and data, which are key components of scientific literacy. At level six, students should be capable of conducting independent research, which requires advanced technical skills to go with their more advanced theoretical understanding, and the ability to design and troubleshoot their own experiments. Developing these skills is essential for students who will go on to careers in biomedical science, research, or related fields[28].

The development of advanced lab skills is not just about technical proficiency. It's also about gaining a deeper understanding of the scientific process. Without a holistic understanding of how these techniques fit into the broader scientific process, students might find themselves competent in performing tasks without truly understanding their relevance. An appreciation of the scientific process promotes critical thinking, a skill that is not only applicable in the lab but across a range of professions. It involves questioning why specific methods are chosen, how data is interpreted, and whether conclusions drawn are reasonable based on the evidence presented. Developing advanced lab skills also requires effective communication. Scientists need to be able to explain their methods, conclusions, and the impact of their work and this requires a deep understanding of the scientific process to accurately and effectively convey complex ideas.

The increase in antibiotic-resistant bacterial infections is a significant global health concern and is a key topic in microbiology modules. The World Health Organization has identified antibiotic resistance as one of the biggest threats to global health and in the face of this challenge, it is essential for students studying biomedical science to understand the factors contributing to the rise of resistance and strategies to combat it.

To further this understanding, we present a lab session based on a real-world scenario: an outbreak of an antibiotic-resistant bacterial infection in a hospital and community setting. This session requires students to integrate their knowledge of epidemiology, bacterial growth and identification, and antibiotic resistance, applying this theoretical understanding to a practical and relevant situation (Table 5.1).

Students are provided with a case report detailing the patients affected, their symptoms, and potential sources of exposure. They then need to determine which information is relevant to the investigation, promoting critical thinking and problem-solving skills. This task encourages students to think like epidemiologists, sifting through data to identify key factors that may contribute to the source and spread of the outbreak.

In preparation for the lab activities, students are asked to review lecture notes on antibiotic resistance and other relevant topics. This not only solidifies their understanding of these topics but also reinforces the relationships between them. Understanding the growth and identification of bacteria, for example, is intrinsically linked to understanding how and why certain bacteria may develop resistance to antibiotics.

This lab session serves multiple purposes. It provides students with an opportunity to apply and integrate theoretical knowledge from different areas, develop critical thinking and problem-solving skills, and gain an appreciation for the complexities and challenges associated with managing antibiotic-resistant infections. The ultimate aim is to prepare students for future careers, where they may be required to tackle similar real-world problems.

In terms of the assessment for this activity, students prepare a report outlining their diagnosis, recommendations for treatment and infection control and the route of the infection. This type of report allows students to showcase a broad range of skills and knowledge and serves as more than just a summary of the lab work; it's an integrated document that combines theoretical understanding with hands-on experience.

Table 5.1 Outline of the activity

Section	Details
Epidemiology and patient data	Students are provided with a case report of an outbreak of an antibiotic-resistant infection in a hospital and community setting. The case report includes information on the patients affected, their symptoms, and potential sources of exposure.
	Students are then asked to identify which information is relevant to the investigation and why in order to demonstrate critical thinking.
	Students should review lecture notes on epidemiology, bacterial growth and identification, antibiotic resistance, and antibiotic resistance profiling to prepare for the lab activities.
Sample handling	Samples of various types are provided in the lab session (blood, urine, respiratory secretions, wound exudate, and environmental surfaces). These can be provided as raw samples/swabs or as agar plates made from the samples.
Microbiological analysis	A range of identification tests are carried out both standard microbiological techniques (Gram stains, selective and differential growth media, API/ biochemical tests) and antibiotic resistance profiling can be carried out. Students are provided with a booklet of the potential tests available, and they should demonstrate critical thinking by justifying which tests to use and why
Molecular analysis	Molecular identification tests will be carried out. PCR and sequencing/electrophoresis can be used for species identification and PCR can also be used for the identification of antibiotic resistance determinants.
Diagnosis	Students combine the results of the lab activities with the patient reports and epidemiological data to produce a justified conclusion regarding the causative species behind the outbreak.
Treatment and infection control	Students should make justified recommendations for suitable treatments and highlight important aspects of infection control
Tracking	Students should produce a report outlining and justifying the source and spread of the infection.

The Diagnosis section provides an opportunity for students to exhibit not just their technical knowledge but also their intellectual depth. In this section, students are tasked with outlining and justifying their diagnostic process, starting from the initial observations and ending with the final diagnosis. The objective here is twofold: to demonstrate a mastery of diagnostic methods and to articulate the reasoning that underpins their choices. Students are expected to elaborate on the lab techniques they employed to arrive at their diagnosis. However, the emphasis isn't solely on the 'what' but also on the 'why'. For instance, if a student chooses to use PCR for DNA analysis, they should explain why this method was more suitable for their specific case compared to other methods like culturing or immunoassays. This provides an opportunity for students to showcase their understanding of the advantages and limitations of various diagnostic tools, as well as their applicability in different scenarios. Beyond the technical aspects, the Diagnosis section should also delve into the interpretative skills of the students. They should discuss how they analysed the data from their tests, what patterns or anomalies they observed, and how these findings led them to their final diagnosis. This is where their critical thinking skills come into play. Students should be encouraged to question their own results, consider alternative explanations, and even discuss any uncertainties or limitations in their diagnostic process. This section should also reflect the students' ability to integrate information from multiple sources. For instance, how did the case report influence their choice of diagnostic tests? Did the symptoms described in the report point them towards specific conditions that needed to be either confirmed or ruled out? This level of integration demonstrates not just technical proficiency but also a more complex problem-solving ability.

The Recommendations for Treatment and Infection Control section requires students to transition from diagnostic reasoning to therapeutic planning and public health strategy. This section should not only be a list of treatments, it should be a comprehensive blueprint that addresses the multi-faceted challenges posed by antibiotic-resistant bacterial infections. Students are expected to recommend specific antibiotics or other treatments based on their diagnostic findings. However, the complexity of antibiotic resistance necessitates that they go beyond merely naming a drug. They should explain the rationale behind their choices, taking into account factors such as the bacteria's resistance profile, the patient's medical history, and potential side effects of the treatment. This allows students to demonstrate their grasp of pharmacology, particularly the mechanisms of action of different antibiotics, their pharmacokinetics and pharmacodynamics, and how these factors influence treatment efficacy. However, treatment is only one part of the equation. Given the public health implications of antibiotic-resistant infections, students must also outline a robust infection control strategy aimed at preventing further spread of the bacteria. This could involve recommendations for isolation procedures, sanitation measures, and even community education initiatives. Students should draw upon their understanding of epidemiology and public health to craft these recommendations, demonstrating an awareness of how individual treatments fit into broader public health goals. Students should consider the practicalities of implementing their recommendations as well. For example, are the recommended antibiotics readily available, and are they cost-effective? Is the infection control strategy feasible given the resources of the healthcare facility in question? These considerations add another layer of complexity to the task, requiring students to think critically about the real-world implications of their recommendations.

The Tracing the Route of Infection section is a practical application of skills that are vital for anyone entering the field of biomedical science or public health. It requires students to don the hat of an epidemiologist, using a data-driven approach to unravel the complexities of how the antibiotic-resistant bacterial infection spreads. Students are expected to meticulously sift through the case report data, cross-referencing it with their lab results to identify potential patterns or clusters of infection. This could involve mapping out the timeline of symptom onset among different patients or analysing the geographical distribution of cases to identify potential hotspots. The aim is to pinpoint where the infection likely originated and how it propagated, whether through person-to-person transmission, environmental factors, or other vectors. Students must also explain the reasoning behind their conclusions, showcasing their ability to interpret data and make logical inferences. For example, if they suspect that the infection spread through contaminated medical equipment, they should provide evidence that supports this hypothesis, such as the presence of the bacteria on similar equipment or a correlation between the use of specific equipment and infection rates. This level of detail not only demonstrates their analytical skills but also their understanding of the scientific method, as they form hypotheses and test them against the data. This section will also reflect the students' ability to integrate diverse forms of information. They might need to consider patient histories, the chronology of reported cases, and even the genetic characteristics of the bacterial strains involved, as revealed by their lab work.

Conclusion

The emphasis on practical skills within biomedical science degrees is not just a necessary component of the curriculum; it is a fundamental pillar in shaping competent and versatile biomedical scientists. This focus on hands-on laboratory skills, combined with theoretical knowledge, equips students with a comprehensive understanding of biomedical science, ensuring they are well-prepared for their future careers. The progressive development of these skills, from basic laboratory techniques to advanced analytical methods, reflects a deliberate and structured approach to education in this field. By gradually building their competencies, students gain not only the technical proficiency required for laboratory work but also develop critical thinking, problem-solving abilities, and a deeper understanding of the scientific process. This holistic approach to learning develops a more profound appreciation of the intricacies of biomedical science, enabling students to apply their skills and knowledge in a variety of professional contexts.

The integration of practical skills with theoretical learning demonstrates the real-world applicability of the curriculum. This approach not only reinforces the students' learning but also enhances their engagement and motivation by showing the relevance of their studies to real-life scenarios. The integration of ethical practices, safety procedures, and effective communication, including the maintenance of thorough lab books, further instils a sense of responsibility and professionalism in students. These aspects are crucial in preparing them not only as skilled technicians but also as conscientious and ethical members of the scientific community.

The importance of practical skills in biomedical science education transcends the acquisition of technical abilities. It involves the cultivation of a well-rounded, ethically aware, and critically thinking scientist. This comprehensive approach to education is needed to prepare students for the challenges and opportunities of a career in biomedical science and beyond, ensuring they are not only competent in their technical abilities but also adaptable, innovative, and ethical in their professional conduct.

References

1. Gliddon CM, Rosengren JR. A laboratory course for teaching laboratory techniques, experimental design, statistical analysis, and peer review process to undergraduate science students. *Biochem Mol Biol Educ.* 2012;40(6):364–371.
2. IBMS. *Criteria and Requirements for the Accreditation of BSc (Hons) Degrees in Biomedical Science*; 2020.
3. IBMS. *Criteria and Requirements for the Accreditation of MSc Degrees in Biomedical Science*; 2020.
4. Subject Benchmark Statement - Biomedical Science and Biomedical Sciences. Accessed September 25, 2023. https://www.qaa.ac.uk/the-quality-code/subject-benchmark-statements/subject-benchmark-statement-biomedical-science-and-biomedical-sciences
5. Herreid CF. *Start with a Story: The Case Study Method of Teaching College Science.* NSTA Press; 2007.
6. Potkonjak V, Gardner M, Callaghan V, et al. Virtual laboratories for education in science, technology, and engineering: A review. *Comput Educ.* 2016;95:309–327.
7. Brockbank A, McGill I. Facilitating reflective learning in higher education. Published 2007. Accessed May 5, 2023. https://books.google.co.uk/books?hl=en&lr=&id=S3Ir9ZcHFn8C&oi=fnd&pg=PP1&dq=value+of+reflective+learning&ots=QtIsSbfa68&sig=t4Evrtne_H5m9ny5kjJnEW5wcNo
8. Akçayır G, Akçayır M. The flipped classroom: A review of its advantages and challenges. *Comput Educ.* 2018;126:334–345.
9. Hunt L, Koenders A, Gynnild V. Assessing practical laboratory skills in undergraduate molecular biology courses. *Assess Eval High Educ.* 2012;37(7):861–874.
10. Gobaw GF, Atagana HI. Assessing laboratory skills performance in undergraduate biology students. *Acad J Interdiscip Stud.* 2016;5(3):113.
11. Staver JR. Constructivism: Sound theory for explicating the practice of science and science teaching. *J Res Sci Teach.* 1998;35(5):501–520.
12. Kolb DA. *Experiential Learning: Experience as the Source of Learning and Development.* FT Press; 2014.
13. Macaulay C, Cree VE. Transfer of learning: concept and process. *Soc Work Educ.* 1999;18(2):183–194.
14. Ericsson KA, Krampe RT, Tesch-Römer C. The role of deliberate practice in the acquisition of expert performance. *Psychol Rev.* 1993;100(3):363–406.

15. Trullàs JC, Blay C, Sarri E, Pujol R. Effectiveness of problem-based learning methodology in undergraduate medical education: A scoping review. *BMC Med Educ.* 2022;22(1):104.
16. Biggs J, Tang C. *EBOOK: Teaching for Quality Learning at University.* McGraw-Hill Education (UK); 2011.
17. Ambrose SA, Bridges MW, DiPietro M, Lovett MC, Norman MK. How learning works: Seven research-based principles for smart teaching. *The Jossey-Bass Higher and Adult Education Series.* 2010;301. https://psycnet.apa.org/fulltext/2015-38684-000.pdf
18. Ghanat S, Garner D, Wittman T, et al. Assessing Students' Metacognitive Skills in a Summer Undergraduate Research Program. In: *2022 ASEE Annual Conference & Exposition.* peer.asee.org; 2022. https://peer.asee.org/assessing-students-metacognitive-skills-in-a-summer-undergraduate-research-program.pdf
19. Boud D, Molloy E. Rethinking models of feedback for learning: The challenge of design. *Assess Eval High Educ.* 2013;38(6):698–712.
20. Fennell RC. Teaching for understanding at university: Deep approaches and distinctive ways of thinking – By Noel Entwistle. *Teach Theol Relig.* 2011;14(3):287–288.
21. Stieff M, Werner SM, Fink B, Meador D. Online prelaboratory videos improve student performance in the general chemistry laboratory. *J Chem Educ.* 2018;95(8):1260–1266.
22. Hattie J, Biggs J, Purdie N. Effects of learning skills interventions on student learning: A meta-analysis. *Rev Educ Res.* 1996;66(2):99–136.
23. Robertson C Linking laboratories to the lecture. *APS April Meet Abstracts,* 1997:I4.01:14–01.
24. Jones SM, Edwards A. Online pre-laboratory exercises enhance student preparedness for first year biology practical classes. *Int J Innov Sci Math Educ.* 2010;18(2). https://openjournals.library.sydney.edu.au/CAL/article/view/4641
25. Basit FHM, Zulfiqar S, Noor S, Huo C. Examining multiple engagements and their impact on students' knowledge acquisition: The moderating role of information overload. *J Appl Res High Educ.* 2021;14(1):366–393.
26. Smetana LK, Bell RL. Computer Simulations to Support Science Instruction and Learning: A critical review of the literature. *Int J Sci Educ.* 2012;34(9):1337–1370.
27. Milanovic I, Eppes T, Sweitzer F. Progressive curricular structure for STEM programs. *Kosmas.* 2009;3:14.
28. Rakhmonkulov FP. Organization of practical and laboratory activities in the educational process. Published 2019. Accessed May 11, 2023. http://www.idpublications.org/wp-content/uploads/2019/11/Full-Paper-ORGANIZATION-OF-PRACTICAL-AND-LABORATORY-ACTIVITIES-IN-THE-EDUCATIONAL-PROCESS.pdf

Part III

Innovative pedagogical approaches in biomedical science education

6 Designing authentic learning practices for mid-degree biomedical science students

Kathryn Dudley and Tara Sabir

Authentic assessment

As a degree programme, biomedical science has the challenge of meeting the requirements of graduates who wish to pursue a diverse range of careers. Some graduates of biomedical science programmes wish to pursue a career as a Biomedical Scientist within the National Health Service (NHS) or private healthcare systems and require a specific set of knowledge and skills. Some graduates wish to pursue a career in industry or academia or to pursue further postgraduate study with a view to entering a masters degree, postgraduate medicine or the physician's associate programme. This makes curriculum design and delivering authentic learning practices for students with a range of postgraduate aspirations difficult. One of the greatest challenges for programme teams is to accurately replicate the time and workload pressures associated with working in a laboratory environment within healthcare, industry or academia, whilst also acknowledging that these challenges may vary according to the field.

Delivery of authentic learning practices requires an accessible curriculum that interests and engages students, regardless of their career aspirations and allows them to develop the knowledge and skills required to obtain graduate employment. These authentic learning practices should reflect professional practice and allow the development of a range of transferrable skills, professionalism, an ability to follow defined protocols, bioethics and an understanding of personal responsibility. One key element of biosciences programmes, including biomedical science, is that graduates develop their laboratory skills through exposure to practical laboratory techniques, following standard operating procedures (SOPs) within a laboratory environment as well as developing an understanding of health and safety within the laboratory and ways to manage risks safely.

The theory-practice gap

There is a recognised theory-practice gap amongst graduates, related to the divide between theoretical ideals generated in academic environments and the expectations of professional practice[1]. Graduates from degree programmes

DOI: 10.4324/9781003383994-10

are not always well prepared for their professional role, and authentic learning practices are important in addressing this. The theory-practice gap has been described extensively across a range of degree programmes in healthcare, including nursing, paramedic science, pharmacy and medicine. In nursing, this gap is greatest for newly qualified professionals due to the physical separation between academic studies and clinical practice which results in difficulties relating theory to practice[2,3]. In biomedical science, this gap is likely to be greater because not all students complete a placement during their studies and therefore are not exposed to clinical or industrial working environments during their course, with many students only gaining laboratory experience from their practical classes. Due to the presence of the theory-practice gap amongst a range of healthcare professions, it is likely to be present for students aspiring to careers as Biomedical Scientists who have not completed a clinical placement.

One strategy for addressing the theory-practice gap is to encourage students to complete a placement during their degree programme. The benefits of placements for students and their future employability are well recognised for the development of transferable skills, better performance in final year studies and the ability to obtain graduate employment within the placement organisation[4-6]. Placements also provide students with real-world experiences and a range of practical skills that are relevant to their future careers. This can help to reduce the theory-practice gap and ensure students are better prepared for their graduate roles. Effective degree programmes develop a range of transferable skills, including communication skills, team working skills and critical thinking which are essential for the future employability of graduates[7]. Often, laboratory experience is required when applying for graduate roles and a lack of experience in a professional laboratory makes obtaining graduate employment challenging[7]. For this reason, biomedical science graduates need sufficient exposure to authentic experiences during their degree programme.

Transferable skills and employability skills should be embedded within curriculum design to ensure that students are well-rounded graduates who will add value to their employer's organisation upon completion of the course. To achieve this, authentic learning practices are required to ensure that students have a good understanding of the clinical, academic or industrial working environment at graduation. Strategies to reduce the theory-practice gap include exposure to the workplace through placement opportunities, the inclusion of practitioner and researcher academic staff on biomedical science programmes to provide real-world experiences and skills to students[8], as well as maximum exposure to working in a laboratory setting through taught practical sessions. Students should be prepared with realistic expectations of the working environment through fostering skills such as professionalism, time management skills and personal responsibility. Where these skills are embedded within the curriculum, it should be made clear to students why these expectations are in place and how this will benefit their future employability.

In addition, students who are seeking employment within healthcare as a Biomedical Scientist should receive input from Health and Care Professions Council (HCPC) registered staff who can effectively manage their expectations and help students understand the real-world applications of the role. This is important to ensure students are adequately prepared for practice and have a good understanding of their chosen graduate role.

Case-based teaching

For those students who aspire to graduate positions within healthcare, case-based teaching can provide an invaluable opportunity for exposure to authentic learning practices which are closely aligned to their future careers. Case-based teaching is a popular method of teaching in the field of healthcare, and it can be used effectively to support student learning[9,10]. This method encourages students to learn through group discussion facilitated by an educator[11]. It requires students to apply their knowledge and analytical skills to realistic scenarios and make complex decisions, requiring a more active learning style than traditional didactic lectures. As a result, case-based teaching increases knowledge, embeds key skills in critical thinking and problem solving and develops transferrable skills such as collaborative learning and communication, whilst encouraging reasoning and decision-making[12–15]. These transferrable skills are essential for those students wishing to pursue a highly skilled graduate career in industry, academia, healthcare, or those wishing to practice as a Biomedical Scientist. In addition, interactive case-based teaching sessions allow for key lecture concepts to be revisited if it becomes evident that there is a lack of understanding amongst the cohort and time should be factored in when planning the session to allow for this.

To actively participate in a case-based teaching session, students need to have sufficient underpinning scientific knowledge to be able to engage with the session[11]. Even if students have attended the preceding lecture session, there is no guarantee that they have engaged sufficiently to allow them to actively participate in discussions surrounding the case. Case-based teaching sessions are challenging to facilitate in large groups as it is easier for students not to participate[12]. Ideally, case-based teaching sessions should be facilitated in small groups where students interact directly with the facilitator who reveals further information as the case progresses[16]. Students may need to carry out further research to actively participate in a case-based teaching session, in which case access to electronic devices or time to analyse the case information outside of the classroom setting may be beneficial. In the context of authentic learning practices, case-based teaching is highly relevant in the field of biomedical science, but this relies upon students drawing upon their personal and professional experiences and subject-specific knowledge. It is important to recognise that those students without exposure to clinical experiences may find case-based teaching sessions more challenging and feel anxious about participation, even if they wish to engage.

Case-based teaching is beneficial for those students who wish to pursue a career in healthcare, particularly as a Biomedical Scientist, because it provides students with real-world experiences of the reasoning and decision-making required within their postgraduate role. This method of teaching is thought to strengthen the link between theory and practice[17], thereby potentially reducing the theory-practice gap. In practical subjects such as biomedical science, purely academic knowledge is of little value unless students can put this into practice through the application of knowledge or hands-on experience. Cases must be well designed to construct appropriate questions and allow for demonstration of the application of basic scientific concepts to real-world situations, which provides a challenge for clinical educators[18]. For those students aspiring to careers in healthcare, case-based teaching develops their understanding of the wider healthcare system and the interaction between various professional roles and disciplines within the multidisciplinary team (MDT). This knowledge can be beneficial when applying for graduate roles.

It is recognised that case-based teaching encourages collaboration and promotes critical thinking and problem-solving skills which are key transferrable skills for a range of professions[19]. Case-based teaching is also beneficial for integrating basic sciences with clinical sciences and promotes the application and retention of knowledge[20]. Students may place higher value on information gained through case-based teaching, perceiving it to be more relevant and are more likely to retain this knowledge in their future careers. Case-based teaching strategies may also help to engage disinterested students, particularly if these methods can incorporate the use of technology to facilitate student participation[21]. Case-based teaching represents an authentic learning practice for students on biomedical science programmes as it fosters a range of transferrable skills and helps to maintain student interest and retention of knowledge by demonstrating the real-world applications of their knowledge and skills. For those students aspiring to careers in healthcare, these skills are essential for their future professional roles. For students aspiring to careers in academia, industry or further study, these activities provide a range of transferrable skills which are applicable in many fields.

Designing a case-based teaching session

For biomedical science educators, the ability to design activities which allow students to develop their critical thinking and problem-solving skills is important[22]. To authentically reflect healthcare practice, case-based teaching sessions should be designed to be interactive and participatory, preferably involving small-group teaching. Groups should identify a spokesperson to give feedback to the larger group. Students should be provided with basic information regarding the case, such as the patient's age and gender and any past medical history but not all of the information included in the case study needs to be immediately relevant to the diagnosis, which is often reflective of a clinical setting where patients present with several different conditions. Students should also be provided with the patient's clinical symptoms and relevant laboratory data with age and gender-appropriate reference ranges provided. If possible, the case study should evolve with further information being revealed through the addition of further diagnostic test results and strategically designed questions to guide the students through the case.

Students should be asked to explain the underlying pathophysiology of the condition and how this aligns with the presenting laboratory data and clinical symptoms to demonstrate a good understanding of the underlying scientific principles of the case[23]. It is also important to consider the alternative diagnoses for a case and encourage students to identify any additional laboratory or clinical tests that would allow a confirmed diagnosis to be made. Whilst designing evolving case studies of this nature can be challenging for the course team, they allow students to demonstrate a critical understanding of a topic, which is required of all graduates of a degree programme. Second-year students on a biomedical science programme should be able to evidence critical analysis of information and the ability to communicate complex information to specialist and non-specialist audiences[24]. This demonstrates that case-based teaching methods are constructively aligned with graduate attributes and allow students to demonstrate achievement of these qualities, meaning that the curriculum is coherently designed and allows students to evidence achievement of the course and module learning outcomes[5]. For those students who aspire to a graduate career within healthcare, case-based teaching provides the opportunity to gain a wider understanding of the integrated nature of the UK healthcare system and how diagnostic testing underpins the work of the wider MDT.

Challenges of simulating the clinical laboratory environment

In the context of a clinical laboratory setting, authentic learning practices require the use of simulated patient data or simulated patient samples to foster the development of analytical and problem-solving skills. Students should be provided with basic case information, including patient demographic information, presenting symptoms and other relevant pathological test results, along with simulated patient samples for analysis. As with case-based teaching methods, these simulated practical experiences allow for the application of critical thinking and problem-solving skills which should be linked back to the underlying pathological principles of a disease. One challenge for course teams is replicating the high degree of automation and the workload pressures which are present in a clinical laboratory. Inevitably, in university practical classes, students will analyse small numbers of simulated specimens, often reverting to manual techniques which are no longer common practice in a clinical laboratory. The challenges of simulating the workload and degree of automation in a clinical environment mean that there may be an increasing reliance on technology to foster these learning experiences and allow students to gain a better understanding of the realities of a clinical laboratory.

To provide a more authentic experience of the clinical laboratory, close collaborations with clinical colleagues, particularly Biomedical or Clinical Scientists within the NHS, should be established to provide a more realistic experience for students. When manual techniques are used, these should demonstrate the underlying principles of automated techniques, which should then be related back to modern larger-scale methods which are reflective of current practice. Technology can also be used to develop more realistic experiences for students, with video technology or simulation exercises used to provide an overview of the pathology laboratory environment[25]. Video technology, with the consent of a local NHS Trust, can also be used to demonstrate the significant workload associated with some NHS Trusts and pathological disciplines and to provide a more authentic experience of working in this environment. Biomedical science students who undertake a healthcare laboratory placement often express that the laboratory environment did not reflect their expectations, highlighting the importance of managing these expectations through authentic experiences that are more closely related to practice.

An evolving job market for the modern-day biomedical scientist

With an ever-increasing number of biomedical scientists qualifying with competitive degrees and entering into an equally competitive job market, it is more relevant than ever to ensure that graduating students are able to gain authentic, transferable lab-based skills as early in the degree programme as possible. As educators, it is also important to keep updating our teaching styles to keep up with current trends in employability. One of those important teaching styles is the introduction of authentic approaches addressing the realities of employment specifically in industry or commercially driven labs, further improving their competitiveness upon qualification[26].

Clinical roles are not the only option for graduating biomedical science students. There is an array of diverse commercial and industry-related job opportunities, which offer interesting and lucrative careers for our graduates. As such it is essential for the modern-day biomedical science graduate to be well-rounded, with a clear understanding of how lab-based skills and training can be transferred into a multitude of roles. Achieving this empowers the graduating student when faced with the challenges of trying to quickly gain employment post qualification. There is evidence that authentic approaches to learning which involve research help students to feel included and benefit from picking up competencies. It is thought that this approach in itself helps improve student mental health and well-being during undergraduate and postgraduate studies[27].

The large spectrum of complex theory taught in biomedical science courses ensures that biomedical science graduates have the opportunity to apply themselves to a wide range of non-clinical job roles. However, the transition to such roles is not always obvious to either the educator, who may have a solely clinical background, and/or the graduate, who may have entered into higher education directly from college or school with no relevant prior work experience.

Since most employers in commercial environments are driven to recruit graduates ready to hit the ground running, employability relies heavily on the authenticity of those skills learned during undergraduate training. If a student is to make themselves attractive to industrial/commercial lab-based roles in this competitive and evolving job market they must understand what it is the employer wants in terms of those skills they have gained during their undergraduate degree[28]

Specifically, the educator needs to directly address lab-based skills such as relevant lab-focused numeracy, transparent data recording and data analysis, time management, independent thinking and self-direction. Additionally, the student needs to understand the principles of accreditation, GLP (good lab practice), GMP (good manufacturing practice) and the roles they, as qualified scientists, play in understanding and signing a risk assessment or formulating it from scratch along with the relevant material data safety sheets.

Authentic approaches to lab-based competencies

The principles and practices of experimental lab work are typically addressed throughout the biomedical science degree, culminating in a research or capstone project in the final year. As students are supervised by active researchers, this project becomes an authentic experience for students and introduces the concepts of self-direction and health and safety as well as lab-related numeracy, data recording and analysis. However, consistency in how these core skills are addressed can vary from one research group to another based on the availability of supporting staff, the type of research being carried out or the type of labs being used and often means that the learning experience, however authentic and valuable, can vary massively from one student to another.

It's also important to note that research projects in the final year of a degree programme within a university environment, whilst being invaluable and an excellent authentic practice, often do not address those key aspects applicable to an industrial or commercial post. Rarely is traceability of data recording embedded or even described and rarely is a student fully aware of the personal responsibility of failing to adhere to the principles of good data recording, nor the different types of accreditation and concepts such as systems validation. Again, unless a student is specifically selecting a year in industry, it is unlikely that an undergraduate would experience or understand the differences and in today's current employability environment, for graduating students, the combined commercial/industry/academic authentic approach, mid degree, is more relevant than ever before[28].

Case study: Authentic learning experiences and targeting key lab-based skills spanning industrial and clinical roles

A graduate's toolbox of knowledge, theory and analytical skills is overflowing through a summation of modules and associated lab practicals by the end of a degree. But which of those tools do they need to employ in that first week in the post as a professional biomedical scientist? Typically, students are faced with the challenges of data recording, basic dilutions, buffer preparations and use of basic instrumentation to include pipettes, pH meters and UV-spectrophotometers in the first few days on the job. Additionally, the ability to address new instrumentation never used before, access and understand SOPs as well as ensure they are covered by the relevant health and safety documents are critical skills needed in those first few weeks. And finally, experimental planning and referring to relevant literature to support the chosen protocols used are equally important.

This approach places a strong emphasis on developing practical skills that are immediately applicable in a lab environment. It also encourages students to become self-reliant problem solvers, capable of navigating challenges without constant supervision. By integrating these elements into the curriculum, the authentic assessment method seeks to produce graduates who are not only knowledgeable but also competent and confident in applying their skills in a professional context[29].

The module, 'Professional Scientific Practice' (PSP) is a level 5 module that aims to develop the independent professional practice by building a platform of skills which would be attractive to an array of biomedical science-related employers. It starts with a unique approach: it simulates the initial days of a professional lab role by assigning students a straightforward research task, devoid of any supplementary materials or guidelines. This setup is deliberately designed to compel students to draw upon the knowledge and skills they've acquired in previous modules. The absence of a structured guide or step-by-step instructions pushes them into the realm of self-directed learning, a crucial skill for any professional setting.

The module's intended learning objectives highlight the key skills and knowledge students will develop and reflect an authentic approach:

1 Plan and manage a laboratory project, including submission of Health & Safety and COSHH documentation.
2 Explain the importance of quality control and quality assurance and their role in good lab practice.
3 Analyse the ethical issues that arise in good lab practice.
4 Demonstrate knowledge of what employability means to an employer.

This is further supported with the assessment where students produce a report based on their lab activities and undertake a lab exam that assesses their competencies. The authentic assessment approach adopted by this module serves as a robust training ground for students, equipping them with the practical skills and self-reliance essential for navigating the complexities of the workforce[30]. Unlike traditional academic assessments that often prioritise theoretical knowledge, this module emphasises real-world tasks that students are likely to encounter in their future professional roles. This focus on practical, hands-on experience is designed to bridge the gap between academic learning and the demands of the job market.

Embedding independent practice and experimental planning

Employers are looking for graduates who hit the ground running, requiring little training and demonstrating reliable lab practices. To prepare students for this, it's crucial to shift away from reliance on lecturers or lab support staff for guidance in experiments and data collection. A student is typically transitioning from a school, teacher-led environment to a university and will, more often than not, rely heavily on approval from the lecturer or supporting staff in experimental planning. A graduating student should be able to plan and time manage their own experimental work without it feeling daunting or indeed a new concept to them. An authentic approach embedded in PSP to encouraging self-led experimental work is the provision of a simple research-related task well within the scope of a mid-degree bioscientist without any supporting material. Over the course of the module and the duration of a single semester, with limited time in the lab, the student is quickly forced to pick up the idea of self-direction. By navigating this process on their own, students are forced to engage more deeply with the task at hand. They must plan their experiments, manage their time, and troubleshoot issues independently. Ultimately, this approach removes reliance on the lecturer or supporting staff and replaces it with the students' own independence and the self-reliance needed to confidently plan and time manage lab-based work[31]. Students who manage to navigate this initial hurdle often find that they are better prepared for similar challenges in a real-world lab environment. They also gain a more realistic understanding of what to expect in their future roles, which can be invaluable in reducing the 'culture shock' often experienced when transitioning from academia to the professional world.

Without this opportunity to fail and repeat on a simple yet realistic task, without support, it is very easy for students to spend the course of a degree blindly following often very complex experimental protocols. Collecting data blindly and data analysing without fully understanding the origins of the protocol's design and inception often means students cannot fully appreciate what it is an employer ultimately wants at the very start. It is important to have the depth of theoretical knowledge but equally developing and researching protocols, instrument use and quality data recording must come first. It is important to change the focus from assessment, to developing the ability to demonstrate and interpret complex theory and with understanding and identifying the importance of finding and evidencing protocols used. This in turn is a much more authentic approach to learning which also focuses the student on what is practically relevant for employability in a commercial/industry-based lab.

Forming a foundation for good data recording, transparency and data trailing

In a commercial or industry-driven setting, experimental data is useless if its basic collection methods and associated errors aren't understood. There are many ways to approach data analysis but the simplicity of good quality data recording and data trailing is equally important. That the data collected must be traceable and completely transparent is difficult for an undergraduate to fully understand, not because it is a difficult concept but more so because we rarely give these competencies full value in teaching. Again, an authentic approach in the lab shifts the focus from theory and instead emphasises the importance of accuracy and accountability in data recording.

PSP uses authentic case studies and debate centred on real-world examples such as the 'Industrial Bio-Test (IBT) laboratories Scandal'[32], to provide an engaging perspective on the consequences of data mismanagement but this however, does not embed the importance of transparency and traceability in experimental data recording in reality. As such, this module develops this further using a basic authentic approach where a simple request, without protocol or supporting material, is followed by an assessment which awards marks for those critical concepts. Is it possible to see the origin of every error? Can the error of every measurement be linked to a particular pipette or UV spectrophotometer? Does the student understand the difference in determining instrument error and analyst error (their own)? Is it clear where and when these measurements were made and ultimately is the data presented clearly authored with a date, time and place. These are simple concepts but if successfully embedded in the foundation of a student's learning create a trustworthy, robust potential employee who can be developed in post. These are exactly the qualities required in those first few days, weeks and months of employment which give the employer confidence in their new recruit. Equally this confidence helps the new employee (our graduates) quickly pick up the relevant training and develop the skills required for the particular post they are employed for.

Building confidence in basic lab-focused numeracy

Within most biomedical science degrees there are of course opportunities for statistical mathematics, biomathematics and aspects of relevant physics covered to some level. However, it is often apparent that some of the simplest numeracy-related skills are difficult for some students to translate into a practical application; it's entirely possible, for example, for a degree to be completed with a student not confident on how to translate an understanding of molarity and molecular weight into the components of a buffer preparation, or how to accurately prepare dilutions or aliquots of samples for multiple measurements. Again, these are the very practicalities that need to be first to hand in the graduate's toolbox. It's not helpful nor encouraging for the new employee to be working all these things out in their first few weeks in a new post.

PSP uses an authentic approach to recreate those first few days at work and allow all the working out to evolve over the course of a module and specifically in a lab environment without any support except what can be drawn from previous modules studied. The point here is to slow those first few hours right down and to focus on those tools and competencies a student would need to engage. Students can perceive this as a 'sink or swim' approach which can be daunting initially for students reliant on being guided through related lab work step by step by lecturers and lab staff. It can take a surprising amount of time for even the brightest of students to work out how to apply their basic numeracy skills to practical considerations and to move away from an instinctive reassurance from those educators around them. However, the reward of students applying their already learnt knowledge and problem-solving independently is invaluable. It is in itself confidence building and in particular that self-perception of confidence is what is required in the first few weeks in a lab-focused job role in order to quickly and competitively progress[33].

Understanding instrument calibration, error and systems validation

One of the key elements of this module is the focus on instrument calibration and understanding errors, which are fundamental aspects of any lab work. Students are given the responsibility to calibrate basic lab instruments and to identify what constitutes an acceptable range of error for each tool. Authenticity in learning here leans heavily on those topics which are relevant in GLP whilst in employment. Anyone entering into a post which is commercial or industrial should be aware of the importance of instrument calibration and systems calibration and therefore the idea of error. Again, not riveting information for the burgeoning biomedical science graduate but essential for quality scientific experimentation and therefore one of those critical tools of understanding all our graduates should have at the end of their degree.

Instrument calibration is perhaps the most authentic task that a student can be asked to undertake. It is not interesting, it is not complex, but it is a genuine way of testing a student's understanding of error, where error differs from instrument to instrument, what percentage is deemed acceptable and also the idea of transparency. The appreciation that percentages of error differ from one manufacturer to another is important for a student to understand. Being transparent is more important than demonstrating no error at all. As such the simple request of identifying errors on the most basic of tools within the lab and learning how to correct this or at the very least record it is an authentic task for a student which would directly relate to the quality of data produced and recorded in post. Again, each of these authentic requests/approaches relies heavily on providing no information at all to the student but allowing them to work it out themselves with a very light supervision to ensure progress[34]. Staff provide minimal guidance, allowing students the freedom to navigate the complexities of calibration and error identification on their own. This lack of direct oversight is intentional; it mimics the conditions students are likely to encounter in a professional lab, where supervisors may not always be available to provide immediate answers. By requiring students to figure things out independently, the module aims to cultivate a sense of self-reliance and problem-solving ability. It's a learning strategy that may initially seem risky, but the rewards are manifold. Students not only gain a deeper understanding of the technical aspects of lab work but also develop the transferrable skills—such as initiative, critical thinking, and self-reliance—that are highly valued in the professional world.

By allowing students to focus on the processes of calibration and characterising error of instruments they are using on a daily basis, as well as identifying their own reproducibility in practice, it is easier to embed the idea of systems validation. Although not necessarily possible to teach using an authentic learning practice, it is much easier for the student to understand the important principles of systems validation between different labs producing the same product for example. Again, understanding how to determine the percentage error on instrument reproducibility and how to correct or improve it through calibration. Understanding where and how to check an instrument manufacturer's calibration method and to maintain that instruments' use are all those tools which are attractive to the employer. They are also the very tools that mean the student appreciates what is involved in systems validation even if they do not experience it during the course of their degree[35].

Evidencing protocols and scientific writing

Another significant component of the PSP module involves students evidencing their experimental protocols. This is an authentic learning task which ensures the student moves firmly away from relying solely on encouragement or confirmation of correctness from the teaching team. Students need to understand that their choice of experimental technique, supported through robust references, is much more important than approval from lecturers and learning officers. It is important that they first rely on their own ideas and support those ideas with peer-reviewed literature, which means that their choice of experimentation cannot easily be criticised by anyone. This encourages the student to realise their own responsibility and gives them an independent direction of practice. Writing protocols concisely takes some effort and thoroughly evidencing these protocol choices with quality references shows the students that they are able to be leaders of their own work. The drive here is to use very relevant competencies to move the student away from relying on the teaching team and to understand that they can direct and lead their own independent practice[36]. By taking the initiative to research, validate, and defend their experimental choices, this module allows students to gain confidence in their ability to conduct independent scientific tasks. This is particularly important as they transition into roles where they may be part of larger research teams, yet still expected to contribute original, well-substantiated work.

The topic of personal responsibility is very difficult to achieve authentically within the constraints of a degree programme. However, it is possible to prepare the students through those competencies already mentioned to ensure that they are at least protected through good practice. Perhaps then personal responsibility becomes evident through good practice in employment. By embedding those critical competencies such as robust numeracy, data trailing, evidencing and transparency the newly employed graduate is at least starting on a good foundation to build on in employment.

Introducing science policy and bioethical debate

This module does not focus only on lab-based skills; another important focus is on ethics in research, through discussions on bioethical principles and debates on current science policies. This serves to enrich the students' academic experience and prepare them for the diverse challenges they will face in their professional lives. Students are introduced to key bioethical principles like autonomy, beneficence, and justice, equipping them to make ethical decisions in their future work. This is particularly important in biomedical science, where research often intersects with human health and well-being. The principles of bioethical thinking are also important to introduce to undergraduate biomedical scientists in order to formulate an understanding of how science policy might be developed. It is an opportunity to introduce ethical thinking theory which allows the student to understand themselves and how their own morality for example, impacts on their professional approach to scientific lab work. In particular, it is possible to use strategic and professional debate to encourage students to understand and reflect on current scientific policy whilst learning to defend their own point of view through evidencing their arguments. Formal debates are embedded in PSP and introducing the idea of building a robust argument evidenced and supported through literature demonstrates the reality of personal responsibility and is an authentic approach to defending a scientific point of view. It is also an opportunity to present scientific views formally in front of their peers which at the very least builds confidence and prepares them for conference-style discussions[37]. The inclusion of these elements in the module fosters a more holistic skill set. Students learn to integrate ethical considerations into their scientific reasoning, a competency that is increasingly important in today's complex research landscape. Graduates are not only technically proficient but also ethically aware and communicatively skilled, making them well-rounded professionals ready to face the challenges of the modern scientific world.

The authentic assessment approach adopted by this module serves as a robust training ground for students, equipping them with the practical skills and self-reliance essential for navigating the complexities of the workforce[30]. Unlike traditional academic assessments that often prioritise theoretical knowledge, this module emphasises real-world tasks that students are likely to encounter in their future professional roles. This focus on practical, hands-on experience is designed to bridge the gap between academic learning and the demands of the job market.

The authentic tasks are carefully chosen to be directly relevant to the kinds of work students will engage in post-graduation. Whether it's calibrating instruments, understanding error margins, or debating ethical considerations, each task serves as a microcosm of a larger professional responsibility. This ensures that the learning is not just theoretical but immediately applicable, providing students with a toolkit of skills and competencies that they can carry into their professional lives. The module also incorporates elements of peer-reviewed research and ethical considerations, further enriching the learning experience. Students are encouraged to validate their experimental protocols through scholarly references and to engage in debates on bioethical principles and current science policies. This not only deepens their academic understanding but also prepares them for the kinds of discourse and ethical decision-making they will encounter in their professional roles.

The approach of this module offers a comprehensive preparation for the workforce. By focusing on real-world tasks and encouraging independent problem-solving, it ensures that students are not just academically equipped but also practically trained and mentally prepared for the challenges and responsibilities they will face in their professional roles.

Conclusion

The implementation of authentic assessment in biomedical science education is a critical and forward-thinking response to the evolving demands of the professional world. This approach recognises the diversity of career paths available to graduates and seeks to provide them with a comprehensive educational experience that bridges the gap between academic theory and real-world practice.

The challenges inherent in designing and delivering a curriculum that meets these needs are significant, yet they are essential to adequately prepare students for the varied landscape of professional opportunities. The strategic incorporation of case-based teaching, lab-based competencies, and real-world scenarios, alongside the emphasis on transferable skills and employability, serves to cultivate a learning environment that is not only intellectually stimulating but also pragmatically relevant. This relevance is crucial in ensuring that graduates are not just knowledgeable in their field but are also adept at applying this knowledge in practical, real-world settings. Developing critical thinking, problem-solving skills, and an understanding of ethical practices within the curriculum should not be missed either. These aspects are vital in equipping students to navigate the complexities and responsibilities of their future roles, particularly in a field as ethically charged and socially impactful as biomedical science, and their inclusion in the curriculum ensures that graduates are well-prepared to contribute effectively and responsibly in their chosen careers.

Finally, the commitment to authentic assessment in biomedical science education reflects a broader educational philosophy that values real-world applicability and lifelong learning. By preparing students not just for their immediate post-graduation roles but also for a career characterised by continuous development and adaptation, educators in this field are setting new standards for excellence in science education. The move towards authentic assessment in biomedical science is a necessary evolution in education, one that promises to produce graduates who are not only academically proficient but also practically skilled, ethically minded, and ready to face the challenges of the modern professional landscape.

References

1. Zieber M, Wojtowicz B. To dwell within: Bridging the theory-practice gap. *Nurs Philos.* 2020;21(2):e12296.
2. Monaghan T A critical analysis of the literature and theoretical perspectives on theory-practice gap amongst newly qualified nurses within the United Kingdom. *Nurse Educ Today.* 2015;35(8):e1–7.
3. Greenway K, Butt G, Walthall H. What is a theory-practice gap? An exploration of the concept. *Nurse Educ Pract.* 2019;34:1–6.
4. Gallacher DCS. Learning beyond the classroom: Biomedical science. In: *University of Huddersfield Employability, Enterprise and Citizenship in Higher Education Conference*; 2012. https://www.researchgate.net/publication/259502751_Learning_beyond_the_classroom_biomedical_science_students'_narratives_of_volunteering_and_developing_employability_skills
5. Yorke MKPT. Embedding employability into the curriculum. Accessed September 26, 2023. https://www.advance-he.ac.uk/knowledge-hub/embedding-employability-curriculum
6. Brooks R, Benton-Kupper J, Slayton D. Curricular aims: Assessment of a university capstone course. *J Gen Educ.* 2004;53(3/4):275–287.
7. Demaria MC, Hodgson Y, Czech DP. Perceptions of transferable skills among biomedical science students in the final-year of their degree: What are the implications for graduate employability? *IJISME.* 2018;26(7). Accessed September 26, 2023. https://openjournals.library.sydney.edu.au/index.php/CAL/article/view/12651
8. McEwen L, Haigh M, Smith SJ, Miller A. Real world experiences? Reflections of current and past students on practitioner inputs to environmental taught masters courses. *Planet.* 2003;6:18–22.
9. Giacalone D Enhancing student learning with case-based teaching and audience response systems in an interdisciplinary Food Science course. *High Learn Res Commun.* 2011;6(3):1.
10. Aluko A, Rana J, Burgin S. Teaching & learning tips 9: Case-based teaching with patients. *Int J Dermatol.* 2018;57(7):858–861.
11. Eseonu O, Carachi R, Brindley N. Case-based anatomy teaching: A viable alternative? *Clin Teach.* 2013;10(4):236–241.
12. Mostert MP. Challenges of case-based teaching. *Behav Anal Today.* 2007;8(4):434–442.
13. Doran J, Healy M, McCutcheon M, O'Callaghan S. From beyond the grade: Reflections on assessments in the context of case-based teaching. *Ir J Manag.* 2011;31(1):3.
14. Gauthier G, Lajoie SP. Do expert clinical teachers have a shared understanding of what constitutes a competent reasoning performance in case-based teaching? *Instr Sci.* 2014;42(4):579–594.
15. Zheng Y, Li J, Wu Q, Wu Y, Guo M, Yu T. Study on the application of case teaching method in the cultivation of master of professional clinical surgery. *Creat Educ.* 2018;09(02):272–279.

16. Gravett S, de Beer J, Odendaal-Kroon R, Merseth KK. The affordances of case-based teaching for the professional learning of student-teachers. *J Curric Stud.* 2017;49(3):369–390.
17. Hudson JN, Buckley P. An evaluation of case-based teaching: Evidence for continuing benefit and realization of aims. *Adv Physiol Educ.* 2004;28(1–4):15–22.
18. Peiman S, Mirzazadeh A, Alizadeh M, et al. A case based-shared teaching approach in undergraduate medical curriculum: A way for integration in basic and clinical sciences. *Acta Med Iran.* 2017;55(4):259–264.
19. Rybarczyk BJ, Baines AT, McVey M, Thompson JT, Wilkins H. A case-based approach increases student learning outcomes and comprehension of cellular respiration concepts. *Biochem Mol Biol Educ.* 2007;35(3):181–186.
20. Malau-Aduli BS, Lee AY, Cooling N, Catchpole M, Jose M, Turner R. Retention of knowledge and perceived relevance of basic sciences in an integrated case-based learning (CBL) curriculum. *BMC Med Educ.* 2013;13:139.
21. Donkin R, Askew E. An evaluation of formative "in-class" versus "E-learning" activities to benefit student learning outcomes in biomedical sciences. *J Biomed Educ.* Published online 2017. http://downloads.hindawi.com/archive/2017/9127978.pdf
22. Suwono H, Pratiwi HE, Susanto H, Susilo H. Enhancement of students' biological literacy and critical thinking of biology through socio-biological case-based learning. *J Pendidik IPA Indones.* 2017;6(2):213–220.
23. Conti CR. Case-based teaching and learning. *Clin Cardiol.* 2006;29(1):1–2.
24. Qaa. UK quality code for higher education. Part A: Setting and maintaining academic standards. *The Frameworks for Higher Education Qualifications of UK Degree-Awarding Bodies.* Published online 2014.
25. Chen H, Kelly M, Hayes C, van Reyk D, Herok G. The use of simulation as a novel experiential learning module in undergraduate science pathophysiology education. *Adv Physiol Educ.* 2016;40(3):335–341.
26. Harvey L New realities: The relationship between higher education and employment. *Tert Educ Manag.* 2000;6(1):3–17.
27. Babco EL, Jesse JK. Employment in the life sciences: A mixed outlook. *Bioscience.* 2005;55(10):879–886.
28. Steiner CJ. Teaching scientists to be incompetent: Educating for industry work. *Bull Sci Technol Soc.* 2000;20(2):123–132.
29. Ornellas A, Falkner K. Enhancing graduates' employability skills through authentic learning approaches. *Skills and Work-Based ....* Published online 2019. doi:10.1108/HESWBL-04-2018-0049
30. Mayne LV, Choate JK, Zahora T. A pathway towards a holistic skills framework in biomedical sciences. In: *Higher Education Research and Development Society of Australasia Annual Conference.* Vol 6. asnevents.s3.amazonaws.com; 2015. http://asnevents.s3.amazonaws.com/Abstrakt-FullPaper/22607-22607Mayne%20et%20alHERDSA2015%20.pdf
31. Chickie-Wolfe, Louise A., Smith Harve, Virginia. Working with Students to Promote Independent Learning. In: Chickie-Wolfe, Louise A., Smith Harve, Virginia (Eds.) *Fostering independent learning: Practical strategies to promote student success,* Guilford Publications.
32. Rosner D, Markowitz G. "Ashamed to Put My Name to It": Monsanto, industrial bio-test laboratories, and the use of fraudulent science, 1969–1985. *Am J Public Health.* 2023;113(6):661–666.

33. Aithal PS, Kumar PM. Approaches to confidence building as a primary objective in postgraduate degree programmes. *Int. J. Appl. Eng.* Published online March 22, 2018. Accessed October 6, 2021. https://papers.ssrn.com/abstract=3147016

34. Magnusson J, Zackariasson M. Student independence in undergraduate projects: Different understandings in different academic contexts. *J Furth High Educ.* 2019;43(10):1404–1419.

35. Cramer JM, Hamilton PT. An internship may not be enough: Enhancing bioscience industry job readiness through practicum experiences. *J Microbiol Biol Educ.* 2017;18(1). doi:10.1128/jmbe.v18i1.1248

36. Sanchez JM. Are basic laboratory skills adequately acquired by undergraduate science students? How control quality methodologies applied to laboratory lessons may help us to find the answer. *Anal Bioanal Chem.* 2022;414(12):3551–3559.

37. Labov JB, Huddleston NF. Integrating policy and decision making into undergraduate science education. *CBE Life Sci Educ.* 2008;7(4):347–352.

7 Effective student-centred assessment and feedback methods in biomedical science

Jess Haigh and Donna Johnson

Assessment design

When designing our assessments, the first thing we need to consider is what is the assessment for. Constructive alignment has had a major impact on higher education curriculum development[1]. It is an outcomes-based approach where outcomes are defined prior to teaching and assessments are then designed to allow students to achieve the stated outcomes[2]. As well as promoting the deeper learning approach, constructive alignment is also designed to increase clarity in expectations. Increased clarity in terms of student expectations has been linked with increased perceptions of competence, more enjoyment and increased effort and the inclusion of teaching activities and assessments aligned more obviously with the Intended Learning Objectives (ILOs) also increases effort and enjoyment. It has also been suggested that course design using constructive alignment may increase student motivation[3].

With this in mind the best place to start with assessment design is our learning objectives, they outline the learning goals of the module and are pitched at a level suitable for the module level. From the ILOs we can get our keywords, describe, discuss etc[4] and these will inform the structure of the assessment questions. We should also consider if we will be assessing all the ILOs in one assessment or more. Once we have this in place, we can then focus on the specific context of our assessment questions. This is going to be driven by the goal of the ILOs – demonstrations of knowledge or competence[5].

Scaffolding and sequencing

We can set students up for success by designing a thoughtful course assessment path that means students can develop skills at each step of their course that prepare them for later assessments[6]. Scaffolding involves designing assessments throughout the curriculum with each one focused on developing a specific skill that will be required in future assessments. By focusing on building skills one at a time and then incorporating previously learned skills students are less likely to feel overwhelmed as cognitive load is reduced[7]. Sequencing is the process of arranging those scaffolded assessments throughout the curriculum

DOI: 10.4324/9781003383994-11

such that each one provides the skills necessary to complete future assignments. Together this means that knowledge and skills are built over the course to prepare students for success in future assessments. This process requires collaboration among teaching staff such that assessments are harmonious across each semester and that all students regardless of their path have the opportunity to develop the same skills.

The notion of scaffolding and sequencing should be explained to students from the beginning of their course. It is important that they understand the concept of practising individual component skills and that they will be working towards integrating in the future. It goes without saying that any assessment must assess the ILOs of the module, when introducing an assessment it is important to make clear both how the assessment relates to the ILOs as well as the skills that they will develop. Following on from this, assessments that will use previously developed skills should be highlighted. By making the links clear, the students can see the relationship between previously developed skills and how they can use those in new more complex task. It also means they can use the feedback from the previous task to strengthen their next piece of work that uses those same skills.

Table 7.1 shows a simple example of scaffolding and sequencing where early assessments tend to focus on one or two skills and these same skills are utilised together in subsequent assessments in years 2 and 3. When assessment briefs are shared with students, these should contain information on the skills developed so they can look back through past assessments and find the relevant ones to aid in their current task.

Another aspect that can be built into this structure is formative assessments, whether these take the format of full drafts or smaller elements that will contribute to the larger assignment, they provide an opportunity to generate feedback and improve. Formative assessments should be introduced in the same

Table 7.1 Scaffolding assessments

Academic year	Assessment type	Example task	Skills developed
1	Group poster	Presentation of experimental findings	Teamwork, communication skills, visual representation of data
1	Written	Data processing exercise	Data analysis
2	Group oral presentation	Critical evaluation of literature via podcast	Teamwork, literature searching, critical analysis, oral communication
3	Capstone project	Dissertation and poster presentation	Data analysis, written communication, literature searching, critical analysis, oral communication, visual representation of data

manner as summative assessments in the sense that skills developed within the assignment are clearly signposted to students such that they are cognisant of the attributes they are working on and aware of which skills they are improving on from the feedback received. It can also be explained to students that partaking in formative assessments builds other important skills such as self-regulated learning and self-motivation[8]. Throughout scaffolding and sequencing it is important to always be clear about all skills developed in any assessment and to highlight transferable aspects.

Inclusive assessment design

In any course the student population is diverse, coming from a range of backgrounds and arriving at university with differing levels of knowledge and confidence in their ability. Therefore, we need to ensure assessments are inclusive. We can do this by being mindful of inclusive assessment design, providing detailed assessment briefs and providing adequate opportunities for clarification to put all students on a level playing field.

The assessment brief should detail what they need to do, what ILOs are being assessed, which skills will they develop and what percentage of the module mark it accounts for and it should also contain a rubric. A successful brief enables students to spend less time working out what is required and more time completing their assignment. Inclusion of a rubric clarifies what it takes to achieve their desired grade, though it is important to familiarise students with how these are used. The brief should be shared both as an accessible document and during a taught session to give a written and verbal explanation. After introducing an assessment to students, they should be given the chance to ask questions.

Interactive activities during assessment briefing and follow-up sessions are a useful aid to enhance student understanding of requirements and expectations for assessments. This might take the form of marking exemplars, peer or self-marking drafts or Q&A drop-in sessions to stimulate discussion. A guided draft marking session gives students the opportunity to engage with the rubric. There is a risk of plagiarism and collusion with peer marking so this should only be utilised if student topics differ sufficiently, but it can be useful for them to see how others have approached the assignment[9]. Self-marking a draft allows students to directly query whether what they have produced fits the brief and where they can improve sections to aim for more marks. Students can also submit a full or partial draft to gain feedback from the instructor, but class size and assignment length may affect whether this is feasible. Building in formative opportunities in the assessment process allows students to feedforward on comments, identify strengths and weaknesses and provides learning opportunities to better prepare and equip them for the summative assessment. Of note, the timing of formative assessment is crucial, ample time must be given for students to process and act upon feedback before the final deadline. It can also be useful to provide an optional session where common mistakes seen in formative submissions are highlighted and further discussed such that students can avoid repeating. This lends itself to inclusive assessment design as it means both personalised and generalised formative feedback is delivered in written and verbal formats, and so is accessible and inclusive of many student needs.

Other simple strategies for ensuring inclusive assessment design include giving sufficient time between the briefing and deadline such that students have ample time to complete the work. Alongside this, being cognisant of other course deadlines and where possible spreading these out across the semester such that students are not overloaded.

An element of choice

Another aspect of inclusive assessment design is building in an element of choice[10]. Much like the notion of scaffolding and sequencing this should be built up over each year of the course to prevent students becoming overwhelmed. To begin with this can take the form of students' choosing a topic for their assignment from a pre-prepared list, for example choosing a disease to focus on. This allows students to choose something that interests them and so they are more likely to engage and be motivated to learn (ref). If giving student's a list of options it can be a good idea to limit how many can sign up for each topic in an effort to limit potential collusion, especially in more creative assignments where students may be tempted to copy each other's ideas.

The next step in building in choice is to allow students to choose a topic for an assignment without giving a defined list of options. This means students really can choose a topic that is meaningful to them. Students may require more guidance with this format, as without limits they can feel overwhelmed by all the options. Often this format requires more input from teaching staff (ref), this can be through discussion sessions to help direct students or there may need to be approval of topics to ensure that student choices are appropriate for the assignment. We do not want to set the students up for failure at the first hurdle by allowing them to choose topics that do not actually fit the assessment brief. Topic approval will depend upon class size, for smaller groups it is possible to run an in-person session or small group meeting to discuss and approve topics. For larger groups an online system might be better suited, virtual learning environments include a journal option which can be used to submit topics privately and then the teaching staff can give feedback through online comments until the topic is approved.

A slightly more complex way to introduce an element of choice is to allow students to choose the method in which they are assessed. This aids in inclusivity of assessment as students are able to opt for an assessment style that they feel best suits their skills and it can improve confidence in their ability to achieve the learning outcomes. It is preferable to limit choice to two to three assessment modes otherwise there is a risk of inadvertently increasing stress for some students and increasing workload where they need to read over briefs and marking schemes for each mode. Some students, especially in earlier higher education years, may not understand their own strengths and weaknesses when it comes it academic study. During the assessment briefing the skills required for each mode should be discussed along with examples of those skills in use so that students can be guided towards the best option for them.

Building in assessment choice in these ways increases student engagement with assessment as well as interaction with the teaching staff. Allowing the students to be involved in assessment design in this way can improve academic integrity as they can choose a topic that is meaningful to them and this gives them a sense of ownership and voice[11]. It also improves the translational skill of decision making and allows students to actively recognise their interests and strengths.

Reflection

Providing time and space for reflection during assessment deepens student learning and enhances their metacognitive knowledge of their own learning styles and experiences in preparation for future use[12]. Metacognition here refers to the student thinking about and assessing their own understanding, learning process and performance during assessment. Reflection requires retrieval, elaboration and generation of new information, and through this improves the robustness of learning[13].

More specifically, asking students to reflect on their learning experience during an assignment allows them to consider any issues that arose and how they overcame them to complete the assessment. They can also identify strengths and weaknesses, allowing them to maintain a record of these and to signpost to themselves the skills they have developed. Reflection aids students in retaining knowledge and being able to transfer learning to new contexts[12]. They can also reflect upon the application of the assignment and the skills within it to highlight the authenticity of the assessment in terms of real-world application. It can be helpful to inform students of these benefits such that they can see the value in reflective activity and also share your own motivation for asking them to reflect. By assigning a proportion of marks to the reflection this encourages students to invest their time and put real thought into the activity[14].

Assessed reflection can take the shape of a short reflective note or summary (verbal or written) at the end of a specific assignment or a longer piece like a learning journal that includes entries throughout the semester in relation to a module. Students can struggle with reflective tasks be it due to a lack of understanding of what is being asked or feeling like they need to share overly personal information when it comes to identifying weaknesses. This can be overcome by promoting metacognition throughout a module using short exercises asking students to critically analyse their own learning experience, either at the end of class or following a formative assignment[15]. This gets the students used to considering their learning process and importantly prepares them for the reflective portion of their assessment. It is also essential to provide clear assessment criteria for the reflection portion of the assignment and explain this during the briefing.

What is feedback?

The purpose of academic feedback is to help students understand their strengths and areas for improvement, to support their learning and development, and to motivate them to continue learning[16]. Feedback can be an important tool for helping students understand how they are progressing and for identifying areas where they need to focus their efforts.

Effective feedback should be timely, specific, and actionable, and should be provided in a way that is constructive, supportive, and objective. It should be based on clear criteria and standards, and in an ideal world, should be tailored to the individual needs and abilities of each student.

In order to get the best out of feedback there are a few things to consider. We should be using a range of different assessment types; these will look at different skill sets and enable different elements of feedback to be provided. We should be providing formative opportunities to help students develop their skills during the learning process. Formative opportunities guide students in identifying their strengths and weaknesses and adjust their learning and assessment preparation accordingly. An important aspect to go alongside formative assessment and feedback is self-reflection. Students should be encouraged to reflect on their feedback and produce plans as to how to make the most of it. A useful document to have here is a feed-forward worksheet. Students can use these to identify where they lost marks and what they should keep an eye out for in future assessments as well as seeing where they did well.

As staff, we likely spend a considerable amount of time producing feedback for our students, however, there often appears to be a disconnect between our perceptions of feedback, its format and usefulness and what our students think about it. A recent questionnaire on feedback given to our biomedical science masters students shows a good understanding of what feedback is and why it is important, but some students still report that they don't use their feedback to improve future assessments and don't consider written feedback to be important overall. There was also some confusion about what formative feedback was though students highlighted the importance of being given opportunities to submit drafts. The responses to this questionnaire suggest some approaches we can take to improve the use and perceptions of feedback in our students. It is a good idea to include feedback information in our induction and module introduction sessions, as well as a dedicated session to go through formative feedback.

In the induction sessions we can give general information and clarify important terms, as well as emphasise the importance of feedback. In our module introductions we should be talking more specifically about the feedback opportunities and format for the specific module/assessments. Here we can also go through how we want the feedback to be used. Activities will be useful here, students can be given a piece of feedback and produce a feed-forward sheet for example, to show them more practically what they should be looking for in their feedback. We can also talk about how we use feedback in our work, a useful example here is how we use reviewer's comments to improve work for publication.

Probably the most important delivery of feedback in a module setting will be that provided for drafts, so where possible, a dedicated feedback session should be provided. This could be in a class session or in shorter one-to-one meetings. Providing sessions like these are the best way to promote engagement with the feedback, they also give students the opportunity to ask questions and clarify their understanding. It is a good idea to use activities in these sessions if they are held in class, as students may be reticent about asking questions in front of their peers.

How do we deliver feedback?

While there are multiple ways we can provide feedback to students the most likely formats will be dialogic or written comments.

Written feedback is the most common type of feedback. Written feedback gives us the opportunity to be quite detailed in our comments and as it is generally delivered online, can be read and digested at the students' preference and pace. It can also benefit those that have some anxiety around receiving feedback as it is often easier without face-to-face interactions. Having written comments allows a record to be kept of the feedback, meaning that it can be referred back to at later timepoints and used in conjunction with other feedback for reflection.

One of the key disadvantages of written feedback is that it can be time-consuming to produce and may only be skimmed by the students. We have no real way of assessing engagement with the feedback and it can be impersonal. Unless it is combined with opportunities for further clarification, it can also be confusing for students and so not used to its full potential.

Written feedback in isolation is unlikely to deliver in terms of engagement and use by the students. It should be used in conjunction with activities designed to promote engagement with it, such as the production of feed-forward plans or reflective pieces, particularly when it is being used for formative purposes. An alternative to written feedback is the use of dialogic feedback where it is given verbally face-to-face, either in person or increasingly in online meetings. Dialogic feedback enables immediate clarification of feedback because students can ask questions then and there. It can be better at promoting engagement and understanding because students are involved in a dialogue with staff about their work and the feedback. It is more straightforward to personalise and explore understanding more deeply using dialogic feedback because we can also provide feedback on students' understanding of the work and the feedback. Having face-to-face meetings with students has the additional benefit of developing more meaningful relationships between staff and students which can promote an environment where students are more likely to seek help when they need it outside of the feedback process.

There are many advantages of dialogic feedback but these need to be weighed against some significant disadvantages. All forms of feedback can be time-consuming but dialogic will definitely take the most amount of time and is very difficult to scale up while remaining sufficiently personal and in-depth. It might not be right for some students, particularly if they are anxious or shy, if feedback in this format is difficult or uncomfortable then it is likely to be considerably less effective.

A further consideration is that it is vital that staff have the necessary skills to provide good feedback in this format. We must be able to ask the right questions, read non-verbal cues when assessing understanding and be able to actively listen to our students. We need to be able to deliver feedback in a way that is clear and constructive, particularly if we need to give feedback on work that is far from the requirements. People can take feedback very personally, especially if they have worked hard on something that doesn't meet requirements and so we must balance getting the right information across while also not discouraging our students.

Because of its more detailed nature, dialogic feedback is particularly useful for providing formative feedback, however, it works best when used alongside written feedback. The best approach would be to provide written feedback, give students time to read and reflect on this and then follow it up with a dialogic feedback session. By following this approach, we can ensure that students are fully engaged with the process and more likely to get the most benefit from it.

This approach is fantastic if we have small classes or multiple staff teaching on a module but what happens if we have large classes? It's not an easy task to provide detailed written feedback on 150 draft essays let alone following each of these up with a meaningful face-to-face meeting and then marking summative assessments on top. There are a few strategies we can use to make life slightly easier.

In most cases, the online platforms we use to mark assessments have the facility to store and use standard phrases. Often the mistakes students make are similar enough that these standard phrases will be useful, especially for more standard considerations such as spelling and grammar. These can be time-consuming to set up but will decrease time in the future. Platforms are also increasingly introducing automatic feedback for things like spelling and grammar so by checking these options in the assessment set-up will save more time, though the use of this information would need to be covered in introduction sessions with the students first. If we take advantage of the automated tools available to use it will free us up for providing more detailed feedback on the more complex elements of the work.

Because the specific mistakes and misconceptions are often fairly common, some care can be taken with explaining these in teaching sessions and provides an opportunity for the provision of more general feedback that can be provided to the whole group via written or dialogic methods. A document or short video going over the more common issues is going to save considerably more time compared to explaining these each time they turn up in a piece of work.

We can set up online questions with model answers provided as feedback. Students can then attempt a question and then compare their answer against the model one to see what they got right and wrong. This has the added benefit of requiring engagement with and reflection on the process from students. Again, the initial set up will be time-consuming but then can be used repeatedly with only minimal updating, can be largely hands off and is easily used in in-class sessions with large groups.

A further approach is to use peer feedback, though this will need time setting aside in class to carry out and adequate time to set up and prepare the students for what they should be looking for and the type of feedback they should be providing. Care must be taken to avoid any chance of bias and lack of objectivity amongst student groups in order for the feedback to be useful. If peer feedback is implemented properly there are some key benefits such as increased engagement and collaboration among peers, improved communication, and increased ownership of learning[17].

Evaluation of assessment and feedback

With every assessment that we design, we should go through an evaluation process to make sure that it is fit for purpose. We should consider the assessment before students do it and then again afterwards. We can then feed this information into monitoring processes and make any necessary adjustments in time for the next cohort.

To start the evaluation process, we need to outline the purpose of the assessment, is it formative and meant to guide students or is it summative and meant to measure student's understanding of a topic? It is important to have this information in place at the start because it will guide the rest of the evaluation process. Next we need to consider the validity and reliability of the assessment – does it measure what we say it measures and will it do this consistently? We should focus on the specific components of the assessment we are measuring and ensure this is reflected in the marking criteria, for example if we're measuring critical thinking then we should prioritise this in the mark allocation and focus less on generalities like spelling and grammar. We should also be evaluating on the basis of fairness, we need to make sure that an assessment is accessible to all our students taking it. We need to ask if it will advantage or disadvantage a particular group of students, for example if an assessment uses complex language or terminology that hasn't been taught, English Language Learners or students with lower language proficiency may be disadvantaged. Finally, we need to make sure an assessment is aligned with the ILOs for the module. The positive impacts of aligning assessments to the ILOs are well documented and this leads to improved performance and enhanced learning[18].

Before we release the assessment to students, it is also worth considering the method of feedback. While time consuming it is generally preferable to provide feedback through both a rubric and either detailed written or dialogic feedback. Does the assessment offer opportunities to provide this type of feedback in a way that students can use to develop skills for future assessments and will you have sufficient time to provide it? If not, it's a good idea to think more about how the assessment is designed with this more of a focus.

Evaluation should continue after the students have submitted their work. At this stage we can consider the marks – are they all clustered together at the top end of the marks range (too easy?), at the bottom range (too hard?) or is there a good spread showing the assessment effectively differentiates between students who have mastered the material and those who have not? This means the assessment is challenging enough for high-achieving students while still being accessible to lower-achieving students. A good distribution of marks may also suggest that the assessment is fair. If only a certain group of students are doing well, while the rest are not, it may indicate a bias in the assessment.

Student feedback is an important component of assessment evaluation too so we should include specific questions about this in the student module evaluations. With this information we gather multiple perspectives on an assessment that will help us to understand more about what worked or didn't work with it.

Evaluating the feedback we provide is less straightforward. Providing feedback is a nuanced process that involves not just the content of the feedback, but also the way it is delivered and used by the students. One way to evaluate feedback is by assessing changes in student performance. If students improve in areas highlighted in the feedback, it suggests that the feedback was effective. Student's opinions on feedback and information about how they use it can also form part of the module evaluations and we can use this information to guide how we deliver feedback and its content.

Self-reflection and peer review are key tools in the evaluation process. We can consider whether we feel confident in our ability to provide effective feedback, whether we have enough time and resources to provide good feedback, and whether we feel our feedback is having a positive impact on student learning. If we also observe each other's feedback practices we can identify areas of best practice and get constructive feedback on what we are doing. This can be a valuable way to share best practices and improve feedback quality.

Case study: Student engagement with assessment and feedback

One of the more frustrating aspects of assessment and feedback from a staff perspective is the feeling that students are not engaging fully with the process. Students are also frustrated with the process, reporting that marks were felt to be unfair and that marking criteria were difficult to interpret and apply[19]. So how do we approach improving this? Research suggests that clarity in rubrics and tailoring of feedback is most effective at improving engagement[20].

In our Medical Biotechnology module (level six), we have implemented a multifaceted approach to assessment and feedback (Table 7.2). This module is worth 20 credits and has two assessments – a set of questions associated with analysis of data collected in lab sessions and an exam with a seen section comprised of an essay-type question and an unseen section based around data analysis and interpretation. Students are introduced to the assessments in the module introduction session and further assessment information is provided in the module guide and assessment briefs.

The provision of assessment briefs has been useful in increasing student awareness of assessment requirements. In each brief there is information about the deadline, feedback time, ILOs assessed, details of the assessment requirements and the marking scheme. They are a useful source of information for students as all the relevant information is contained within one document. We release these documents before the module starts and then go through each brief in the module introduction session, giving the students an opportunity to ask questions and clarify the requirements.

The coursework assessment gives students an opportunity to present and interpret data that they have collected in the lab, this then prepares them for similarly structured questions in their exam. Preparation for the essay section of the exam is covered in the revision session. In this session, we start with a short presentation about the final assessment and look at the marking scheme to be used for the essay question, then we go through an example question matrix so students have a good way of clarifying their understanding of the exam question. The final activity is to mark two different example essays using the standard marking scheme and produce feedback for the answers.

Table 7.2 Integration of assessment preparation activities in a level 6 medical biotechnology module

Time	Goal	Activities
In module introduction	Introduce assessments	Go through the assessment briefs Go through the marking scheme Q and A session
In lab sessions	Assess student understanding of coursework requirements	Go through the assessment questions
After lab sessions	Support students in learning the data analysis methods	Example data is provided and we analyse the data in class and discuss the results
Revision session	Assess and increase student preparedness for exam	Overview of the marking scheme Students are provided with two example essays (both pass level, one above 70%, one around 45%) Mark them as a class against the marking scheme and model the answerProduce a feed-forward plan

Table 7.3 Example question matrix

	Keyword/Concept	*Details*
Instruction	Discuss	Consider the pros and cons of an issue Compare and contrast Provide evidence in support of your points
Topic	Personal genetic testing	Whole genome sequencing, transcriptomics, genetic testing, diagnosis, prognosis, treatment
Context	Healthcare	Focus on use in/by the NHS, compare to other countries, any differences? What are they and what's their impact?
Focus	Pros and cons	What are the pros/cons Why are they pros and cons What is the impact of each Is this different across different audiences

We consider four aspects of a question in our matrices – instruction, topic, context, and focus (Table 7.3). We then look at the question text and sort keywords into each of the boxes and then add details for each. In our sessions we use the example question 'Discuss the pros and cons of personal genetic testing'. Using this question, the instruction in the text is discussed. The topic is personal genetic testing and we want to look at this topic in the context of healthcare and then the particular focus is on the pros and cons of this technology. For our instruction, we need to discuss so we then go over what is meant by this keyword and what we might expect to do in an answer to a question that includes it. Typically, it will require an in-depth answer that takes into account all aspects of the debate concerning a research topic or argument. Students must demonstrate reasoning skills with this type of question and use evidence to make a case for or against (in this case pros/cons) a research topic. Students are reminded that every time they make a statement they must provide a citation to support it; for example, if they say that the widespread use of PGT is harmful, they should find literature that supports this conclusion and then reference it. Next, we add details to the topic.

The question asks for information about PGT so we would focus there. But PGT is not just one approach to testing so students are made aware that they should talk about the methods used in PGT and also those used in more traditional settings of genetic testing. For the context, we'd start by focussing on healthcare, and here they could talk about why people choose to use PGT. Finally, we consider the focus. The important keywords here are pros and cons. As well as stating and explaining these, students also need to consider things like:

- The impact on different audiences.
- Has it been beneficial for the public?
- Has it made a difference to patient treatment/diagnosis?
- Has there been an effect on clinicians?
- Are there further requirements for extra education or training that make life easier or harder for medical staff?
- How might general genetics education impact whether PGT is good or bad?

This exercise will then be followed up with going over the details for sections of an essay (introduction, main body, conclusion) and the Point, Evidence, Explanation, Link (PEEL) structure for writing paragraphs.

The most useful activity in this session is getting students to mark example answers to our example question using the marking scheme. We provide students with two examples, one that would achieve a mark of over 70% and one that would achieve a mark between 40 and 45%. We use examples with such a mark difference so students can more easily highlight the particularly good parts as they tend to stand out more. For the lower mark essay, there are obvious omissions such as a plan or correctly formatted references as well as less in-depth main body. We find this activity to be particularly useful as it reinforces what we have discussed about the question and the requirements for answering it and helps students to better understand what we look for within each grade boundary and the types of things they should be writing in order to achieve higher marks. Once students have marked their examples and provided feedback, we discuss this as a class and come up with a final mark and set of feedback, we then talk about how this feedback might be used to feed forward into future assessments.

By using this approach to assessment preparation, we have seen consistently good outcomes for our students, not just in terms of the marks they achieve but also in their engagement with the assessment process and their understanding of the importance and utility of feedback.

Overall, the best approach will be to consider assessment and feedback holistically across a course and to embed authentic assessment types where possible. Students should be provided with detailed explanations of each assessment type and a suitable and specific rubric. The format of these documents should be consistent across the course as should the provision of draft opportunities and feedback sessions.

The design of the assessment is crucial in achieving this, but it is equally important to provide appropriate feedback throughout a student's learning journey. There is often dissatisfaction expressed in student surveys regarding assessment and feedback. The long wait times for marks and perceived variability in feedback quality are common concerns. Simultaneously, we as educators often feel frustration regarding the under-use of feedback by students and the challenges associated with the assessment workload.

Conclusion

Producing authentic and effective assessment, especially in a field as diverse as biomedical science, requires a detailed approach. The first step is to carefully consider the assessment design. The goal should be to create assessments that are fit for purpose, accurately measuring student understanding without being onerous to mark. Secondly, it's essential to ensure a mutual understanding between staff and students about the nature of feedback and its intended use. This might involve clear communication about the aims of feedback, supported by teaching sessions specifically designed to cover how to use feedback effectively. Finally, we need to consider how to integrate feedback throughout the learning journey in a way that supports ongoing learning and achievement. This might involve providing formative feedback at multiple stages of the learning process, not just after summative assessments. It could also involve strategies like peer feedback or self-assessment, which can provide additional feedback opportunities and help students develop valuable self-regulation skills.

The ultimate goal is to create an integrated approach to assessment and feedback that enhances learning and achievement for all students, regardless of the subject they're studying.

References

1. Kandlbinder P. Constructive alignment in university teaching. *HERDSA News*. 2014;36(3):5–6.
2. Biggs J Constructive alignment in university teaching. *HERDSA Review of Higher Education*. 1, 5–22. Published online 2014.
3. Stamov Roßnagel C, Fitzallen N, Lo BaidoK. Constructive alignment and the learning experience: relationships with student motivation and perceived learning demands. *Higher Education Research & Development*. 2021;40(4):838–851.
4. Bloom BS, Committee of College and University Examiners. In *Taxonomy of Educational Objectives*. Vol 2. Longmans; 1964.
5. Jackson N, Jamieson A, Khan A. *Assessment in Medical Education and Training: A Practical Guide*. Radcliffe Publishing; 2007.
6. Wilson K, Devereux L. Scaffolding theory: High challenge, high support in Academic Language and Learning (ALL) contexts. *Journal of Academic Language and Learning*. 2014;8(3):A91–A100.
7. van Merrienboer JJG, Kirschner PA, Kester L. Taking the load off a learner's mind: Instructional design for complex learning. *Educational Psychologist* 2003;38(1):5–13.
8. Nicol DJ, Macfarlane-Dick D. Formative assessment and self-regulated learning: A model and seven principles of good feedback practice. *Studies in Higher Education*. 2006;31(2):199–218.
9. Boud D, Cohen R, Sampson J. Peer learning and assessment. *Assessment & Evaluation in Higher Education*. 1999;24(4):413–426.
10. Morris C, Milton E, Goldstone R. Case study: Suggesting choice: Inclusive assessment processes. *Higher Education Pedagogies*. 2019;4(1):435–447.

11. Thibodeaux T, Harapnuik D, Cummings C. Student perceptions of the influence of choice, ownership, and voice in learning and the learning environment. *International Journal of Teaching and Learning in Higher Education*. 2019;31(1):50–62.
12. Jackson N. Developing the concept of metalearning. *Innovations in Education and Teaching International*. 2004;41(4):391–403.
13. Brown PC, Roediger HL III, McDaniel MA. *Make It Stick: The Science of Successful Learning*. Harvard University Press; 2014.
14. Colthorpe K, Sharifirad T, Ainscough L, Anderson S, Zimbardi K. Prompting undergraduate students' metacognition of learning: Implementing 'meta-learning' assessment tasks in the biomedical sciences. *Assessment & Evaluation in Higher Education*. 2018;43(2):272–285.
15. Tanner KD. Promoting student metacognition. *LSE*. 2012;11(2):113–120.
16. Dawson P, Henderson M, Mahoney P, et al. What makes for effective feedback: staff and student perspectives. *Assessment & Evaluation in Higher Education*. 2019;44(1):25–36.
17. Patchan MM, Schunn CD. Understanding the benefits of providing peer feedback: How students respond to peers' texts of varying quality. *Instructional Science*. 2015;43(5):591–614.
18. McMahon T, Thakore H. Achieving constructive alignment: Putting outcomes first. *Quality in Higher Education*. 2006;3:10–19.
19. Graham AI, Harner C, Marsham S. Can assessment-specific marking criteria and electronic comment libraries increase student engagement with assessment and feedback? *Assessment & Evaluation in Higher Education*. 2022;47(7):1071–1086.
20. Jordan S Student engagement with assessment and feedback: Some lessons from short-answer free-text e-assessment questions. *Computers and Education*. 2012;58(2):818–834.

8 The capstone experience
Creating changemakers

David I Lewis

What do we mean by a capstone experience?

Capstones for me are an inspirational, transformative and translational culminating educational experience, where learners bring together competencies gained earlier in their programmes and apply these to a problem, developing new competencies in creating a solution or output for that problem.

They originated in the United States. A high-impact educational practice[1], their purpose is to enable learners to integrate their learning in the US 'pick and mix' system of Higher Education, where learners on the same programme have usually taken very different portfolios of modules or courses. Capstones have traditionally been conservative in nature, an extended essay, a taught seminar series or service learning experience[2] and university educators globally have not made full use of their transformative (massive uplift in competencies) and translational (preparation for the workplace) nature.

Undergraduate and taught postgraduate research projects

Undergraduate and taught postgraduates, particularly in STEM disciplines, have traditionally undertaken a major research project towards the end of their programmes, for undergraduates their Final Year research or Honours project[3-6]. In biomedical science and broader Biosciences, this is normally a laboratory-based, fieldwork or literature project, with the purpose for learners to gain research experience. Some programmes do offer other opportunities, for example, science in schools or enterprise projects, however these are still research projects both in design and purpose[7,8].

It is becoming increasingly apparent the majority of graduates, particularly undergraduates, do not go on to careers in research. We are not addressing the educational or developmental needs of this underserved majority by requiring them to undertake a traditional research project. Instead, educators globally, and across all disciplines, need to re-imagine the purpose, practices, and outcomes of the Final Year, Honours or taught postgraduate project in order to better prepare all learners for the diversity of careers they go into.

DOI: 10.4324/9781003383994-12

The solution is an enhanced capstone project or experience, combining the US capstone experience, where learners gain work experience and develop work-related competencies (knowledge, skills and behaviours)[9], with the UK concept of a research or enquiry project. Any activity can be a capstone, including traditional laboratory-based or fieldwork projects, provided learners are given ownership and responsibility for their project (rather than being research assistants following a defined set of instructions)[10]. Each capstone provides different work experiences and develops different sets of competencies and the idea is that programmes offer a portfolio of capstone opportunities, with learners selecting the one that best addresses their individual developmental needs and/or career aspirations[10]. This provision of a portfolio of opportunities is inclusive as there is something for everybody. It provides the opportunity for every learner, irrespective of background or prior lived experiences, to realise their full academic potential, personal ambitions and goals.

We also need to stop thinking of the project as the end point assessment of a degree programme. Instead, it should be the vehicle to transition learners onto the next stage of their life-long learning journey.

It does require a change of mindset of all stakeholders – learners, educators, Institutions, Professional, Regulatory and Statutory Bodies, employers and Society, and the removal of personal, disciplinary or Institutional 'blinkers'.

Developing changemakers

Ultimately, our goal as educators is to develop Changemakers, graduates who go on to become leaders in their field, equipped with the competencies to be able to make a real difference in the world by contributing solutions to the complex problems facing the world and humankind.

To fully realise this transformative and translational impact of capstones on learner outcomes and futures, educators need to do more than just offer a broad portfolio of opportunities. It is going to require both learners and educators to think beyond their traditional disciplinary and institutional practices and norms, better replicating the workplace in everything they do.

Firstly, there is a need to give learner's ownership and responsibility for their educational experiences and learning, in short '*My course, my future, my capstone*'. To re-imagine relationships, so no longer are there students and supervisors, instead mentees and mentors, with mentors allowing mentees to make mistakes, to reflect on and learn from them, and to apply this learning going forward[11]. Secondly, to shift to learner-centred, community or client-engaged experiential learning opportunities, where, instead of pre-defined projects, teams of learners have a brief or task to complete for a client as you would in the workplace[12]. The 'client' could be virtual or real, a university academic, industry, government, non-governmental or community organisation or any other stakeholder. The teams would, within the resources available, create solutions or outputs for this client-initiated problem. Finally, the outputs or solutions would be assessed, either individually or as a team, using appropriate workplace tasks or activities[13].

A portfolio of capstone opportunities

These client briefs can be sub-divided into three broad themes: research, science or industry-facing and social justice capstone opportunities[10] (Figure 8.1).

Research capstones

Research capstones are designed to provide research experience and develop research competencies for those learners intending to go into careers in research or other careers where research competencies would be beneficial[10,14]. They encompass the traditional opportunities, for example, laboratory-based, fieldwork and critical reviews of the literature, but also other research-based opportunities that educators, to date, have made limited use of, including data analytics, bioinformatics, computational and computational modelling.

Critical to the success of these is putting learners and their educational experience as the primary aim rather than seeing them as an additional pair of hands or source of pilot data for their mentor's research. It requires giving teams of learners experience and responsibility for all stages of the research process, from identifying the research question, creating a hypothesis, experimental design and execution of the research, to data analysis and interpretation[14].

To maximise the learning and the development of competencies that can only be realised through team working, it should be true team working, with all team members being involved in all elements of the research rather than each learner working independently on the same research question.

The key competencies developed include experimental and research skills, experimental design, data mining, analysis and visualisation, numerical and analytical, digital literacy, critical thinking, team working, negotiation, service orientation, planning and organisation[14].

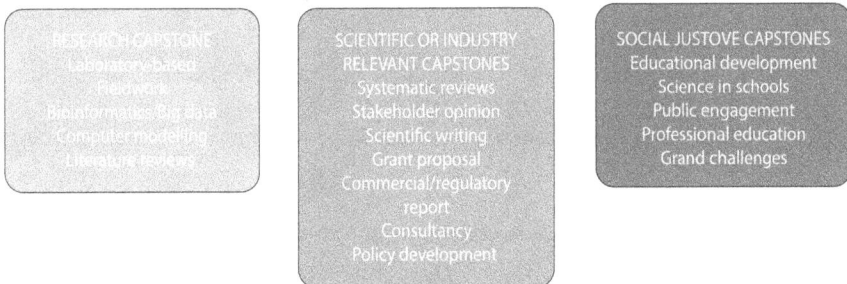

RESEARCH CAPSTONE	SCIENTIFIC OR INDUSTRY	SOCIAL JUSTOVE CAPSTONES
Laboratory-based	RELEVANT CAPSTONES	Educational development
Fieldwork	Systematic reviews	Science in schools
Bioinformatics/Big data	Stakeholder opinion	Public engagement
Computer modelling	Scientific writing	Professional education
Literature reviews	Grant proposal	Grand challenges
	Commercial/regulatory report	
	Consultancy	
	Policy development	

Figure 8.1 A portfolio of capstone opportunities.

Example research questions could include:

- Pharmacology of Legal Highs.
- Behavioural assessment of mouse models of neuro-psychiatric diseases.
- Rapid infection diagnostics to help fight antimicrobial resistance.
- Using the Dementia Platform UK data portal to analyse dementia datasets.
- Pharmacological modulation of identified neuronal ion channels in-silico: Impact on repetitive firing behaviour.

Given that learners are never going to write a traditional dissertation again, the recommended primary output is an academic paper in the style and length (~4,500 words) of a relevant journal in their discipline[13].

Science and industry-facing capstones

Science and industry-facing capstones provide the opportunity for learners to apply their scientific competencies and gain work experience in scientific environments outside of traditional bioscience research[14]. They are ideal for learners who might wish to go into careers in consultancy or involve the creation of business, technical or regulatory reports, public policy or careers where they have to collate, analyse and report information in areas they may not have significant expertise in.

Science and industry-facing opportunities include systematic reviews (with or without meta-analysis), scoping reviews, stakeholder opinions (focus groups, surveys etc.), consultancy, business or technical reports, policy documents, and Grand Challenges reports. See '*Choosing your Bioscience Capstone*'[14] for more detailed descriptions of these opportunities and the enquiry approaches used.

The key competencies developed include information searching, collation and evaluation; communication; numerical and analytical; critical thinking; independent working; use of initiative; planning and organisation; self-management and commercial awareness[14].

Examples of science and industry-facing capstones include:

- Scoping review of an experimental or analytical methodology (Consultancy, Client = Researcher or Analytical laboratory)
- Public attitudes to and knowledge of antimicrobial resistance (Stakeholder opinion, Client = Researcher)
- The importance of S-palmitoylation (Scientific writing of webpage content, Client = Small to Medium Enterprise company).

The suggested written output for science and industry-facing capstone is either a business style report, briefing note or policy document[13].

Social justice capstones

Social justice capstones provide opportunities for learners to work with, or for the benefit of, the community or wider Society[14]. They are ideally suited for learners who wish to go onto careers in education, training or professional development, in the development of educational resources or activities, international development and policy, or careers that require excellent communication skills or involve taking complex information and making it accessible to different audiences (e.g. public engagement, medicine, healthcare, sales and marketing, leadership roles)[14].

The key competencies developed from these opportunities include cultural and societal awareness, empathy, social orientation, communication and creative problem-solving[14].

Social justice capstones encompass a broad range of community-engaged experiential learning opportunities including the development and delivery of educational or professional educational resources and activities (including for schools, implementation into degree programmes or to complement an organisations or communities educational programmes), public engagement activities and Grand Challenges reports. See '*Choosing your Bioscience Capstone*'[14] for more detailed descriptions of these different opportunities.

Examples of social justice capstones include:

- My Amazing Brain (interactive workshop for use in primary schools)
- Build a Body (ten easy-to-create interactive activities/models for primary school teachers to use to explain how different organs of the body function)
- Re-purposing an aspirin urinary excretion practical (University degree programme)
- Commercialisation of OrthoPure XT (gamification of a PGT medical technology module)
- All you need to know about Statins (patient information leaflet for local GP surgery)
- Creating frugal solutions to the scourge of Malaria (Grand Challenges)

The suggested primary written output for social justice capstones is a reflective e-portfolio.

In the UK, biomedical science programmes may be accredited by the Institute of Biomedical Science (IBMS)[15] and/or the Royal Society of Biology (RSB)[16]. The RSB also accredit programmes across the broader Biosciences[16]. The IBMS require capstones that include critical thinking, data analysis and interpretation, they do not all have to be laboratory-based research capstones[15]. All three themes described above are acceptable to the RSB[16]. For current details of the formats of capstone acceptable to each Accrediting Body, visit their degree accreditation webpages.

Appropriate, authentic assessments

Historically, the principal assessment tool or approach for both undergraduate and taught postgraduate research projects has been an extended dissertation. However, few learners, even those going onto research degrees or careers in research, are ever going to write a dissertation again[13]. As we broaden our portfolios of capstone opportunities, if we stick with dissertations, there is going to be an ever-increasing disconnect between the activity and how it is assessed. What is needed are alternative assessment approaches that represent activities or outputs undertaken in the workplace, are better aligned to learner's individual capstone opportunities, and are capable of assessing the broad range of competencies developed or used[13].

In keeping the capstone concept of preparation for the workplace, we also need to broaden our thinking, no longer viewing the final year or taught postgraduate project assessment as an endpoint or culminating assessment, rather as an approach to facilitate a learner's transition into the next stage of their career journey.

Whatever assessment approach(es) are offered, it is critical to give learners ownership and responsibility for their assessment, for them to select the approach most suited to their capstone format, but also the one which best showcases what they have achieved and their competencies to future employers, to us as educators, and most importantly, to themselves. So, for example, we could suggest those undertaking laboratory-based or other traditional research capstones create a 4500-word academic paper instead of a dissertation[13]. We could suggest commercial or technical reports are assessed using a business style report format, comprising of an executive summary, introduction and brief, evidence-driven main body, conclusions and SMART recommendations[17].

In adopting these authentic approaches, we have moved from assessing learning to the much more impactful learning through assessment. Learners are gaining workplace relevant experiences and developing competencies through completing the assessment.

We also need to 'de-risk' both these assessment approaches and capstones themselves, by providing opportunities to complete similar assessments and activities in earlier years of their education.

Challenges and solutions

Moving from traditional laboratory-based final-year research, honours or masters projects to offering a broad portfolio of capstone projects can be daunting, requiring both learners and educators to lose their historical disciplinary or Institutional blinkers, and to step outside of their comfort zones. Below are some of the challenges faced, not only in biomedical science but across all disciplines, and our suggested solutions, based on our experiences.

The capstone concept itself

For some educators used to traditional disciplinary research projects, even the name 'capstones' raises concerns. Some institutions are sticking with calling them capstones, while others are calling them 'entrepreneurial projects' or final year projects. In the end, it doesn't matter what they are called, it is the adoption of the capstone concept (opportunities that provide work experiences and develop competencies) that matters. Whatever they are called, it should not include the word research as this sends the message that they have to follow traditional, hypothesis-driven scientific research approaches

Selling the concept to learners and educators

Learners, once they are made aware of the huge positive impact on their educational experience, outcomes, and futures, fully buy into the capstone concept. For educators, it is a marketing exercise – a need to evidence the impact on learners, demonstrate their academic equivalence to traditional undergraduate and taught postgraduate research projects, and that we are not replacing these but broadening our portfolio of other enquiry-based opportunities to better match the career destinations of all our graduates. We need to showcase what's in it for them, changing mindsets so that learners are viewed as a valuable resource rather than a burden, who, through their capstones, can make excellent and creative contributions to all areas of their activity, not just research. Finally, the decrease in workload, including assessment load, compared to traditional research projects is a key benefit, as is their optional nature – they only have to offer capstones in areas they are comfortable with.

Academic equivalence

Educators unfamiliar with capstones commonly question their academic equivalence to traditional research projects. In biomedical science, we have very defined or conservative ideas of what research and data are. Research is traditionally undertaken in laboratories, with the outputs of these activities, our data. This issue does not exist, for example, in creative disciplines where a wide range of totally different activities constitute 'research', with a similarly broad range of outputs. All capstones require a scholarly approach, which may not replicate traditional biomedical science research, but is a research approach used in other disciplines across your Institution. Similarly, information doesn't have to be solely the outputs of scientific investigation. The solution is to broaden our thinking and/or use broad terms that encompass all activities such as enquiry-based learning and information.

Historically, the laboratory-based research project has been the Gold Standard within biomedical science, with a misconception among both learners and educators that capstones are an easy option, not as academically challenging as laboratory-based opportunities. This could not be further from the truth. Learners having to assimilate knowledge in areas they are unfamiliar with or use scholarly approaches from outside their discipline provide the same level of academic challenge as working in a biomedical science research laboratory for the first time. They rise to the challenge, particularly if given ownership and responsibility for their learning and experiences, creating outstanding outputs that are most definitely academically equivalent to traditional outputs.

Initially, to demonstrate academic equivalence, it is recommended that a single written output (dissertation or academic paper) be used for all formats, with blind, second marking of the output by an educator who does not offer that format of capstone. As portfolios of opportunities are developed within programmes, and with it, an increasing mismatch between activity and assessment, learners should be offered a choice of primary output, extending the capstone concept of ownership and choice beyond the opportunity and into its assessment[13]. Robust assessment rubrics should be created (or adopted from other disciplines) that assess the format of written output (academic paper, business report, e-portfolio) rather than the capstone format, with these different rubrics being of a similar structure and format.

Finally, to cement the message, all formats of capstone, including traditional research projects, should be offered within a single module or course. That way, learners and educators view them all as equivalent; no format is seen as the Gold Standard. It also facilitates administration, learners may select different formats of opportunity as their first, second choice etc., and educators can offer different opportunities within the same module

Building a portfolio of opportunities

Once you have taken the plunge and decided to offer capstones, start small. A pilot study. One or two educators collaborating to create one or two new opportunities in an area they have expertise in or are comfortable with, for a few learners. Work with these learners in a collaborative learning partnership[18] so they both undertake the capstone and work with you at the same time to develop the opportunity, for example, producing learner guidance or assessment rubrics.

As programmes progressively develop their portfolios, there is a risk of overwhelming learners with choice, particularly on courses/modules with large numbers of learners and when they are faced with having to choose their capstone project from a long list of individual projects of many totally different formats. Their choices would not be informed, and it would be a resource-intensive administrative nightmare. The solution is to move to Briefs, broadly defined tasks for which teams of learners create solutions to. Multiple teams of learners and mentors would be involved in a single brief, with each team using the capstone approach of their choice to address the brief.

In capstone choices meetings, what each capstone format involves, the experiences and competencies gained, and the broad career opportunities these may lead to, should be clearly articulated. Learners select the choice of brief and describe the experiences and competencies they would like to gain. They are then matched to an opportunity, team and mentor based on this information. This approach is inclusive, unbiased and gives learners input into the allocation process.

As portfolios of opportunities expand beyond traditional research projects, there is a need to provide appropriate scaffolding and support, not only along-side capstone modules, but also in earlier years of degree programmes. Both undergraduate and taught postgraduate projects have a high credit tariff; they are therefore viewed by learners as high-risk. To promote the adoption and equity of experience and outcomes, it is critical to de-risk capstones by providing similar educational experiences and assessments earlier in programmes. Educators also require support. This could include co-mentoring of learners with a more experienced colleague the first time they offer a particular opportunity, co-creation, with colleagues and learners, of new opportunities (Collaborative Learning Partnerships[18]), creation of Communities of Practice, or Team-teaching.

Professional, regulatory and accrediting bodies

Professional, Regulatory and Accrediting Bodies have historically been conservative in approach. However, times are changing. In the United Kingdom, the majority of Quality Assurance Agency (QAA) Benchmark statements have been recently revised[19], all now require the inclusion of Equity, Diversity and Inclusion education, Education for Sustainable Development, and Entrepreneurial Education and Entrepreneurship. The capstone provides an opportunity to embed all of these into programmes. The Biosciences QAA Benchmark Statement now requires a broader capstone rather than a research project[20].

In light of these changes, accrediting bodies are progressively making substantial changes to their own accreditation criteria. The RSB requires the provision of a portfolio of capstone projects (undergraduate) or Period of Practice (masters), where any opportunity, as long as it meets set criteria (including critical thinking, analysis of information and creativity), is suitable[17]. The IBMS permits projects that require critical thinking and analysis of data and refers to several capstone examples that meet this brief in their accreditation criteria[18].

Workload and resourcing

Undergraduate and postgraduate projects require significant resources staff, space and budget. This can be substantially reduced by offering team-based opportunities, non-laboratory based capstones (that free up expensive research and teaching space and lower consumable/running costs), reducing the assessment load (for educators and learners) by replacing the dissertation with more authentic assessments, and focused feedback on drafts, with assessment of final outputs limited to comments on the extent to which they have met the assessment criteria.

Start of a local and global journey

Educators and Institutions globally, not only in biomedical science but in the Biosciences and across all disciplines, are increasingly recognising the inspirational inclusive learner experience that capstones provide, as well as their transformational and translational impact on learners, and are progressively introducing them into their programmes.

Capstones enable learners to realise and showcase their full academic potential, ambitions and goals. They graduate as Global Changemakers, equipped with the work experiences and the competencies to make a difference in the world and to contribute solutions to the complex challenges facing humankind. As educators, we are providing an inspirational, inclusive educational experience for our learners that equips them to succeed in whatever career they go into. They can also make creative contributions, through their capstones, to our own activities. Through Social Justice Capstones, Institutions can engage with the local and global community, thereby realising their civic and societal missions. Employers will be able to recruit graduates with the experiences and competencies required to take their businesses to the next level and to prosper in an increasingly challenging global marketplace. Together, these will realise huge collective benefits for society.

Finally, embrace the capstone concept. Do not be afraid to experiment. Start small, a pilot study, one new opportunity, a few learners and staff, working together to develop the opportunity. Reflect on and learn from your experiences, progressively developing and expanding your portfolio of opportunities.

Case studies: Capstones for biomedical sciences

Capstones enable learners to apply their disciplinary knowledge in different contexts, to explore areas of specific interest to themselves, to gain different work experiences and to develop the specific competencies required for their individual lifelong learning journey. Not every opportunity appeals to, or is suitable, for every learner. It is up to them to select the one best suited for them – the one that best enables them to realise their full potential, goals and ambitions.

Biomedical sciences graduates may go onto careers outside of biomedical sciences laboratories or research. The scientific and other competencies possessed by biomedical sciences graduates are highly valued by employers from many sectors, opening up a broad and diverse range of career opportunities beyond the laboratory for them. Different capstones provide different experiences and develop different competencies, each format better preparing learners for different types of opportunities or sectors. For example, consultancy projects are best suited for learners looking for careers in business including as business leaders, entrepreneurs or management consultants. Public engagement projects prepare students for careers in science communication, education, sales and marketing and community healthcare. The case studies below provide more details of the experiences and competencies developed by different opportunities, and the broad career pathways each can lead to or indeed be a safe space to try out. They also provide details of what each opportunity entails for learners.

Other capstones, not listed, will provide different experiences and competencies, and lead to other non-laboratory or research-based careers. For details of these other opportunities, visit 'Choosing the right Capstone for you'[13].

If your degrees are accredited[15,16], you should also check with your accrediting body, that any opportunity you create is within the scope of their capstone accreditation criteria.

Case study 1: Consultancy

Consultancy activities[13] enable learners to extend and apply their knowledge outside of a traditional biomedical science environment, for example, for a Small or Medium Enterprise, giving them the experience of working in a business or other workplace environment. They undertake activities for their client for which the client lacks the resource(s) or expertise to undertake. The nature of the consultancy varies from client to client and can include, for example, market reports, product placement reports, regulatory requirements, or scoping reviews of methodologies and approaches.

In undertaking these activities, learners gain an insight and experience of the real-world application of science and scientific knowledge in Industry, and also of business and industry work. They gain an understanding of regulation, finance, leadership and management and entrepreneurship and develop additional competencies that can only be gained in a workplace or regulatory environment, for example, discovering, collating, evaluating, storyboarding and reporting information that they are unfamiliar with (e.g. financial, healthcare or regulatory data), entrepreneurial, service orientation and cultural competencies. It enables them to reflect on the broader societal context and the real-world application of science and scientific knowledge. They are an opportunity to realise, for interested students, the QAA Benchmark requirement of the provision of enterprise and entrepreneurial education[19].

The benefits of consultancy capstones extend beyond the learner. They can be critical for SMEs and Start-ups in providing much-needed resource and expertise for specific projects. They contribute to the building of bridges and partnerships between Academics, Institutions and their locality, thereby addressing Institutional civic missions and responsibilities.

Opportunity: Scoping review of the regulations governing the care and use of animals for scientific purposes across Africa.

Brief: The client is an educator who provides professional educational opportunities for individuals involved in the care and use of research animals in Africa. To inform the content of these courses, they require information of the legislation, guidelines and ethical review processes and procedures currently in place in named African countries.

Activity: The team of learners met with the client to agree approach, target audience, objective, purpose and style of the proposed output. They subsequently identified the types and sources of information required to satisfy the client's brief. In this case, national legislation and guidance, and other publically available information sources, with cross-checking against published scientific papers of research involving animals undertaken in each country. This information was collated, and a consultancy report (as previously agreed with the client) created, with conclusions and SMART recommendations that addressed the Brief and their client's business needs[17].

Competencies developed: Information discovery, collation and analysis; communication; creative problem solving; critical thinking; entrepreneurship independent working; use of initiative; planning and organisation; project management; self-management.

Broad career pathways: Careers that require commercial or technical reports, or other defined styles of writing (e.g. consultancy, scientific writing, Regulatory Affairs, policy, clinical trials). Careers where you have to collate, analyse and report, or storyboard, or display graphically information in areas you may not have significant expertise in (e.g. business, marketing, regulation, policy, international development).

Output: Business style report[17] and/or any other output (Briefing note, Standard Operating Procedure, policy document) required by the client.

Case study 2: Stakeholder opinion

Stakeholder opinion[13] capstones involve learners gathering opinions of sections of the community or other stakeholders on issues relevant to their client or their discipline. They can be eye-opening in raising their understanding of the wider societal impact of their discipline, of societal concerns particularly of controversial topics in science, or regulatory, ethical or economic considerations.

Learners undertake in-person or online surveys, focus groups or semi-structured interviews on behalf of their clients (including academics), the outputs, for example, informing research, providing patient and public involvement data, information for funding applications, educational activities, or business activities. They could engage with different sections of the community, healthcare professionals, industry, or other stakeholders, depending on their client's needs. In doing so, they gain cultural and societal awareness and capital.

The benefits of consultancy capstones extend beyond the learner. They contribute valuable information to their client's activities, including, for academic clients, to research, funding applications, and patient and public involvement.

Opportunity: Public attitudes to and knowledge of antimicrobial resistance.
Brief: The client has significant funding for research studies into antimicrobial resistance (this is an example. It could be any area of research within your Institution). To provide the Patient and Public Involvement required by the Funding Body, and to support future grant applications, the client requires information on the attitudes to, and knowledge of, antimicrobial resistance in different sections of the local community.

Activity: The team of learners met with the client to agree on the information required, the approach, the target audience and the required output. They used this information to create both in-person and online surveys on antimicrobial resistance designed to probe the public's knowledge and understanding of the topic. These were disseminated to the required stakeholder communities. The data obtained was analysed, including exploring the themes required by the client (e.g. age, socio-economic background, ethnicity) for differences in opinion. They created a briefing note, with conclusions and SMART recommendations that addressed the Brief and their client's needs.

Competencies developed: Qualitative and qualitative research methodologies; numerical and analytical; digital literacy; communication; service orientation; planning and organisation; independent and team working; leadership; resilience; cultural and ethical awareness and capital.

Broad career pathways: Careers that require interaction and engagement with different sections of the community e.g. social science research, market research, sales and marketing. Careers where you would analyse and use/implement information from stakeholders e.g. sales and marketing, policy development, business, healthcare, consultancy.

Output: Briefing note and/or any other output (e.g. Business style report[17]) required by the client.

Case study 3: Public engagement

Public engagement[13] capstones are community-engaged experiential learning opportunities. They engage learners with their local communities. In doing so, they broaden the public's understanding and appreciation of science, particularly in hard-to-reach communities. It is critical that these opportunities are engagement not communication, a two-way process where learners also learn from the community. It is culturally responsive education, where they are immersed in and learn from different cultures and communities. They develop an awareness and appreciation of society's concerns about science and scientific discovery, multicultural awareness and competencies, and invaluable communication skills. If you can effectively communicate a complex scientific concept to a seven-year-old, you will have no difficulty communicating information to any other stakeholder group or in different environments (e.g. business), a competency that will be invaluable whatever career they go onto. They open learner's eyes to careers and opportunities beyond the laboratory or scientific environments.

Learners are also ambassadors for their discipline, Faculty, Institution and science, building bridges between the Institution and its local community. They are role models encouraging young people to study STEM subjects and consider careers in STEM.

These public engagement activities can take place in any forum, for example, community fetes, community groups, schools, shopping arcades, museums, agricultural shows, music festivals, and for any audience of any age or background. An invaluable opportunity to engage traditional hard-to-reach sections of the community. The harder to reach the community, the more rewarding these opportunities are.

Opportunity: Inspirational science workshops in schools.

Brief: The client, a university educator, seeks to raise awareness of STEM disciplines and careers in STEM with local young people, and to support admissions to their programme. The client requires teams of learners to create and deliver interactive science workshops in local schools and colleges that inspire and engage students.

Activity: Learners engage with teachers within local schools and colleges to agree to topics that both address their needs and align with the national curriculum, or GCSE and A-Level syllabi, the target age groups and the number of workshops required. They used a design and build approach, common in engineering disciplines (lesson plan, evaluate, prototype resources, evaluate, proposed workshop, evaluate) to create their workshop. The evaluations of each stage were provided by focus groups and were used to inform the next stage of the design process. They also form the data for their capstones, as limited data can be obtained from evaluating the live workshops themselves.

The workshops were designed to be highly interactive, with lots of engaging hands-on activities. They were delivered multiple times to different year groups within the same school/college (the core workshop was modified to suit the different age groups) or to different schools/colleges. In all, between 20 and 25 times per workshop. They were delivered to either primary (yr3–6) or secondary (yr10–13) school audiences.

The created educational and supplementary (e.g. lesson plans) were given to the client for use in subsequent outreach activities, shared with the participating schools for use in subsequent years, and uploaded to the University's externally facing outreach webpages.

Competencies developed: Communication; social orientation; empathy; creativity; educational awareness; flexibility and adaptability; use of initiative; planning and organisational skill; self-management; resilience; ethical and cultural awareness and capital.

Broad career pathways: Careers in education or working with the Community or in the development of educational resources/activities. Careers that require excellent communication skills or involve taking complex information and making it accessible to different audiences (public engagement, medicine, healthcare, sales and marketing, leadership roles).

Output: Reflective e-portfolio, public engagement resources and activities, and any other output (e.g. planning documents, lesson plans) required by the client.

Case study 4: Educational resource development

Educational resource development[13] capstones are also community-engaged learning opportunities. The community spans the entire educational spectrum from primary, GSCE, A-Level, undergraduate and postgraduate students to professional education or contributing to the educational activities of community groups or organisations. The activities or resources created are similarly broad from interactive workshops, workbooks, podcasts, and information boards, dependent on the client's needs.

In undertaking these capstones, learners have to apply their disciplinary knowledge to create activities that are appropriate in-depth, detailed and formatted for their target audience. They have to convey complex information in a way that is understandable yet still scientifically accurate. In doing so, they reinforce their own disciplinary knowledge and understanding. They gain experience and competencies in curriculum design, design thinking, storyboarding, scholarship, pedagogical principles and approaches, and qualitative and quantitative evaluation approaches.

Opportunity: Reimagining a salivary secretion practical.

Brief: The client, a university educator, seeks to re-imagine an existing level five practical (could be any educational activity within your programme). They require the team of learners to create an engaging, experimental design-focused mini-project from an existing recipe-driven practical, suggest replacements for outdated approaches and equipment, and digitise the activity by inclusion onto the school's laboratory digital learning platform.

Activity: The capstone team met with the client to discuss their requirements. They ran focus groups with previous level five learners who had participated in the existing practical activity to ascertain their feedback on it and suggestions for change. They discussed practicalities with the technical, learning design and digital support colleagues, and used this information to create a prototype activity. This prototype was evaluated by focus groups, with this information used to create the final educational activity. The created resources, support resources and recommendations for implementation were given to the client, who then introduced the activity into their programme.

Competencies developed: Design thinking; curriculum design; creative problem solving; communication; storyboarding; planning and organisation; qualitative and qualitative research; digital literacy.

Broad career pathways: Careers in education, training or professional development, or in the development of educational resources or activities. Careers that require excellent communication competencies or involve taking complex information and making it accessible to different audiences (e.g. public engagement, medicine, healthcare, sales and marketing, leadership roles).

Case study 5: Grand challenges or UN sustainable development goal capstones

Grand challenges or UN Sustainable Development Goal (SDG) capstones are a novel trans-national community-engaged learning opportunity which provides the opportunity for learners to undertake a deep dive into different cultures and communities. They collaborate digitally with teams of learners in the Global South to create evidence-informed solutions, drawing ideas from both the Global South and Global North to a Grand Challenge or UN SDG relevant to their discipline. This transnational collaborative education experience, where all learners are equally valued and respected, is critical to realise the full personal and professional developmental benefits of this intervention. Each learner bringing different competencies, cultural perspectives and prior lived experiences to the partnership.

The biggest learning from these opportunities is about themselves and others. It is a massive learning experience, opening up their eyes to different cultures and communities, the complex challenges facing humankind globally, but also how their discipline can offer solutions to these challenges. They mature rapidly as individuals, develop global cultural capital and awareness, and become ethically aware.

Opportunity: Creating frugal solutions to the scourge of Malaria.

Lewis DI & *Kwanashie HO. University of Leeds, UK; *National Open University of Nigeria, Nigeria

Brief: The client is a virtual client, a global society. They require frugal solutions (affordable, capable of implementation in the host country or region) to combat the economic, societal, and human and animal health and well-being challenges caused by malaria. The solutions must be drawn from both the Global South and Global North.

Activity: This was a transnational digital educational opportunity involving multi-disciplinary teams of learners from both the University of Leeds and the National Open University of Nigeria working in an inclusive collaborative partnership. After reflecting on the broad theme of their challenge (malaria but could be anything related to their disciplines), the team used a design thinking[21] approach to identify stakeholders, empathise with them, and define and understand the problems and challenges faced by each stakeholder group. At each stage of the process, they used an inclusive 'divergence-convergence' approach – they each reflected independently (divergence) and then combined all their ideas/thoughts together (convergence), excluding nothing, so everybody's thoughts were equally valued and respected. They used this information to focus the direction of their enquiries (e.g. public health, economic, social, disease prevention, regulatory), generating diverse ideas which address the problems or challenges in ways that meet the needs of all end-users and stakeholders. Publically available datasets and other information sources were searched, to provide the evidence to inform the development of these solutions, which were then tested, refined and finalised. At each stage of the Design Thinking process, learners reflected on their learning about themselves and others, and applied this learning to the next stage of the process.

The output was an evidence driven e-portfolio[13] or business-style report[17], with SMART recommendations.

Competencies developed: Design thinking; global cultural awareness and capital; self-awareness; service orientation; empathy; ethical awareness; communication; complex information searching, collation and evaluation; creative problem solving; entrepreneurship; digital literacy.

Broad career pathways: Careers in international development, global health and well-being, policy development, consultancy. Careers that require commercial or technical reports, or other defined styles of writing (e.g. consultancy, scientific writing, Regulatory Affairs, policy, clinical trials). Careers where you have to collate, analyse and report information in areas you may not have significant expertise in (e.g. business, marketing, regulation, policy, international development). Careers that require cultural and ethical awareness and excellent communication competencies (e.g. public engagement, medicine, healthcare, sales and marketing, leadership roles).

Conclusion

The capstone experience emerges as a vital and dynamic element in contemporary higher education, transcending traditional academic boundaries and encouraging a more inclusive, practical, and globally relevant approach. Its evolution from conservative roots in the United States to a more expansive, transformative model reflects a growing recognition of the diverse career paths and aspirations of students. The integration of the US model of work experience and competency development with the UK approach to research and enquiry offers a potent combination, enabling students to gain valuable skills and experiences tailored to their unique developmental needs and career goals. The capstone's potential as a catalyst for change is particularly noteworthy. By reimagining the final year or postgraduate project as a platform for lifelong learning and professional transition, the capstone challenges conventional educational norms. It encourages a shift towards learner-centred, experiential opportunities, blurring the lines between student and professional roles. This approach not only equips students with the necessary skills and knowledge for their future careers but also instils a sense of ownership and responsibility for their learning journey. It can also play a crucial role in developing changemakers – graduates who are not only academically proficient but also possess the creativity, critical thinking, and adaptability to address complex global challenges. By embracing diverse capstone opportunities, students gain exposure to a range of experiences, from traditional research to social justice projects, each fostering different skill sets and perspectives. This diversity ensures that every student, regardless of background or prior experience, can find a capstone that aligns with their personal and professional aspirations.

In essence, the capstone experience symbolises a significant shift in higher education, one that emphasises practical application, personal development, and global engagement. As educators and institutions continue to explore and expand capstone opportunities, they not only enhance the educational experience of their students but also contribute to the broader societal good. By developing a generation of well-rounded, adaptable, and socially conscious graduates, the capstone experience holds the promise of a more innovative, inclusive, and sustainable future.

References

1. Kuh G High-impact educational practices: What they are, who has access to them, and why they matter. Association of American Colleges and Universities. Published online 2008. Accessed October 16, 2023. https://www.aacu.org/publication/high-impact-educational-practices-what-they-are-who-has-access-to-them-and-why-they-matter

2. National Survey of Student Engagement. Engagement Insights: Survey Findings on the Quality of Undergraduate Education – Annual Results 2018. Published online 2018. Accessed October 16, 2023. https://scholarworks.iu.edu/dspace/bitstream/handle/2022/23391/NSSE_2018_Annual_Results.pdf?sequence=1&isAllowed=y

3. Quality Assurance Agency. *Biosciences Benchmark Statement*, 2019.

4. Government of India, All India Council for Technical Education. Accessed October 16, 2023. http://www.aicte-india.org

5. Pharmacy Council of India. The Gazette of India, No. 19, PART III, SECTION 4, Pharm. D. Regulations 2008. Published 10 May 2008. Accessed October 16, 2023. http://www.pci.nic.in

6. Royal Society of Biology. *The Degree Accreditation Handbook*. Royal Society of Biology; 2015.

7. Luck M *Student Research projects: Guidance on practice in the Biosciences.* (Wilson J. ed). Centre for Biosciences; 2008. https://core.ac.uk/download/pdf/18530417.pdf

8. Healey M, Stibble LAA, Derounian. *Developing and enhancing undergraduate final-year projects and dissertations.* Higher Education Academy. Published online 2013. Accessed October 16, 2023. https://www.advance-he.ac.uk/knowledge-hub/developing-and-enhancing-undergraduate-final-year-projects-and-dissertations

9. Ketcham CJ, Weaver AG, Moore JL *(Eds)*. *Cultivating Capstones: Designing High-Quality Culminating Experiences for Student Learning.* Taylor & Francis; 2023.

10. Lewis DI, Bean J, Beaudoin C, Van Zile-Tamsen C, von der Heidt T. Preparing students for the Twenty-First Century workplace. In Ketcham CJ, Weaver AG, Moore JL, eds. *Cultivating Capstones: Designing High-Quality Culminating Experiences for Student Learning.* Taylor & Francis; 2023.

11. Helyer R. Learning through reflection: The critical role of reflection in work-based learning (WBL). *Journal of Work-Applied Management.* 2015; 7(1): 15–27.

12. Kolb DA. *Experiential Learning: Experience as the Source of Learning and Development.* FT Press; 2014.

13. Lewis DI. *Is the Dissertation past its use-by date?* OD&PL University of Leeds. Published May 24, 2023. Accessed October 16, 2023. https://studenteddev.leeds.ac.uk/news/is-the-dissertation-past-its-use-by-date/

14. Lewis DI. *Choosing the Right Final Year Research, Honours or Capstone Project for You. Skills, Career Pathways and What's Involved.* University of Leeds; 2020. Accessed October 16, 2023. https://bit.ly/ChoosingBioCapstone

15. Institute of Biomedical Sciences. *Criteria and Requirements for the Accreditation of BSc (Hons) in Biomedical Science.* 2022.

16. Royal Society of Biology. *The Accreditation handbook.* Royal Society of Biology; 2020.

17. Salford University Library. *Business style reports.* Published online 2019. Accessed October 21, 2023. https://www.salford.ac.uk/sites/default/files/2020–06/Business-Style-Reports.pdf

18. Healey M, Flint A and Harrington, K. *Engagement Through Partnership: Students as Partners in Learning and Teaching in Higher Education.* Published online 2014. Accessed October 16, 2023. https://www.advance-he.ac.uk/knowledge-hub/engagement-through-partnership-students-partners-learning-and-teaching-higher

19. Quality Assurance Agency. *Subject Benchmark Statements.* 2023.

20. Quality Assurance Agency. *Biosciences Benchmark Statement.* 2023.

21. Morgan T, Jaspersen LJ (Eds). *Design thinking for Student Projects.* SAGE Publishing; 2022.

Part IV

Skills development and professional practice

9 Developing key skills in science communication

Donna Johnson

Communication in biomedical science

Biomedical science sits in a unique place within academia, it serves as a source of groundbreaking discoveries and innovations that hold immense potential for human health and well-being, but it also brings an equally important challenge to the forefront: the need for effective communication, which is vital for both teaching and applying biomedical science.

These days, society's health and well-being hinge greatly on science. Issues like a viral pandemic or genetic mutations pay no mind to borders or political lines. However, our collective response to these challenges greatly depends on our understanding and application of scientific knowledge. Effective communication bridges the gap between scientists and policymakers, engages with the general public, and fosters collaborations within the scientific community. The success of these endeavours hinges upon the ability to convey complex scientific concepts in a clear, accurate, and accessible manner. This puts a spotlight on effective communication in biomedical science—it's not just a nice-to-have in biomedical science education, but an absolute must[1]. The advent of social media and online platforms has transformed the landscape of information dissemination, opening up new avenues for scientific dialogue and engagement. However, this technological revolution has also birthed challenges, as misinformation and pseudoscience can easily propagate and influence public opinion. The emergence of echo chambers and filter bubbles further exacerbates the situation, reinforcing existing beliefs and impeding the acceptance of scientific evidence[2]. Dissemination of scientific knowledge is no longer confined to traditional academic channels but encompasses a diverse array of communication modes from journal articles and conference presentations to science journalism and public outreach initiatives, the avenues for science communication have expanded exponentially. However, each medium comes with its own set of challenges and considerations, requiring scientists and science communicators to navigate a complex web of ethical responsibilities, audience expectations, and information accessibility.

In the context of biomedical science education, the significance of teaching effective science communication cannot be overstated. While undergraduate

DOI: 10.4324/9781003383994-14

and postgraduate biomedical science courses typically emphasise the acquisition of technical skills and theoretical knowledge, the art of communicating science often remains underemphasised. Graduates are expected to not only excel in their specialised fields but also possess the ability to effectively convey scientific information to diverse audiences, ranging from fellow scientists and healthcare professionals to policymakers and the general public, yet it is not always a focus for teaching. The consequences of inadequate science communication teaching extend beyond the realm of individual employability. In a society heavily influenced by scientific advancements, the public's perception of science and scientists is shaped by how information is presented and disseminated. The proliferation of misinformation and pseudoscience erodes public trust in scientific institutions and undermines the acceptance of evidence-based knowledge. By equipping students with effective science communication skills, biomedical science courses can contribute to fostering a scientifically literate society that appreciates the value of rigorous research and critical thinking. The teaching of science communication should encompass various dimensions to address the diverse needs of students and future science professionals[3]. It should encompass the development of oral and written communication skills, the ability to distil complex scientific concepts into clear and engaging narratives, and the cultivation of effective science storytelling techniques. Additionally, critical evaluation skills are vital, empowering individuals to discern reliable information from dubious sources and actively participate in debunking misinformation.

Why should we include science communication in our curricula?

The realm of biomedical science is vast, encompassing a wide array of sub-disciplines that combine to inform the complex picture of health and disease. To decipher and contribute to the field, the skill to relay scientific information coherently and efficiently is more than a desired skill; it is vital. Nonetheless, an exploration of current biomedical science courses suggests an unexpected reality—the explicit inclusion of science communication in curricula often finds itself overlooked. This mirrors a stark divergence between expectations and reality; academic institutes envision graduates armed with an intellectual arsenal that can be wielded to articulate complex scientific ideas to a wide array of audiences. In contrast, a palpable lack of formal training in science communication leaves graduates grappling to bridge the gap between knowledge acquisition and its effective communication. This discrepancy, subtle yet significant, carries serious implications, especially when viewed through the lens of employability. Effective communication becomes a passport to varied opportunities, it is a skill that translates complex science into engaging narratives, promotes collaboration and, ultimately, leads to solutions that improve health outcomes. It thus becomes clear that competent science communication correlates strongly with enhanced employability.

In an era marked by unprecedented access to information, an unanticipated problem has emerged: the proliferation of scientific misinformation[4]. Now more than ever, the collective consciousness of society is being manipulated by a barrage of distorted truths, particularly in the domain of science. The ease of online platforms has catalysed the spread of misinformation, with consequential implications on the public perception of science and scientists. These distortions of scientific truth have a significant bearing on public perception of science and scientists. They undermine the credibility of legitimate research, engender scepticism towards the scientific community, and erode public trust in science. When misinformation casts doubt on scientific consensus, it can diminish the public's willingness to support scientific endeavours or adhere to evidence-based recommendations. This scepticism towards scientific truth is detrimental not only to scientific progress but also to society's ability to make informed decisions on critical issues.

The reverberations of this misinformation epidemic underscore the urgent necessity of fostering critical evaluation skills. It is incumbent upon educational institutions and society at large to prioritise the development of these skills, which allow individuals to verify and evaluate scientific information. Being able to discern credible sources, understand the scientific process, and appreciate the nuances of scientific discourse are critical in this age of information abundance. Empowering our students with these skills is not just about combating misinformation—it is about fostering scientific literacy. A scientifically literate society is not easily swayed by untrue claims. It appreciates the iterative nature of science, understands the importance of evidence, and respects the collective wisdom of the scientific community. In the face of rampant misinformation, scientific literacy is an essential line of defence[5].

Teaching strategies

The 'sage on the stage' approach carries with it the weight of tradition. It's a straightforward, instructor-led model where the educator stands as the primary source of knowledge. In this model, students absorb and reproduce the facts and theories presented. The focus here is on the delivery of information from an expert to the learner, often with minimal interaction in between. While this method has been instrumental in laying the bedrock of scientific principles for many students, it's been increasingly subjected to criticism. Detractors argue that it encourages passive learning, allowing students to become mere spectators in their education rather than active participants. The main issue is that while this method may provide students with a wealth of knowledge, it may not necessarily equip them with the skills to communicate this knowledge effectively. It's one thing to understand complex scientific theories and another to explain them in a way that a diverse range of people can comprehend.

This realisation has led to the exploration of alternative educational strategies. It's opened the door to teaching methods that place greater emphasis on interaction and active learning. In these models, students aren't just passive recipients of information. Instead, they engage with the material, with their peers, and with their educators in a more dynamic way. They learn to explain concepts, argue their viewpoints, and respond to counterarguments. In short, they acquire the very communication skills that the 'sage on the stage' approach may overlook.

As we pivot from the traditional model and venture into more innovative methodologies, we find a range of teaching strategies designed to foster science communication. Among them, two particularly promising approaches rise to the fore: case-based learning[6] and project-based learning[7,8].

The case-based learning approach offers students a far more immersive and active educational experience. Here, the primary resource is not a textbook, but real-world examples or cases. These cases, drawn from scientific resources, offer concrete illustrations of abstract principles, making the material more relatable and understandable. The beauty of case-based learning lies in its dual emphasis on comprehension and communication. Students don't only memorise concepts; they dissect them and argue their perspectives with peers. This active engagement facilitates a deeper understanding of the subject matter, and the discussion-oriented setting hones their communication skills. It compels them to articulate complex ideas clearly and persuasively, effectively preparing them for real-world scientific dialogue.

The project-based learning technique takes a slightly different route towards the same goal. In this approach, students are given a research project to work on from start to finish. It's like a simulation of the scientific process, and students are the lead researchers. This method moves students out of their comfort zone, requiring them to tackle a research question, conduct experiments or gather data, analyse results, and then communicate their findings. This hands-on experience provides an authentic taste of scientific research, demanding not just comprehension of scientific principles but also effective presentation of their results. By managing and presenting their own project, students gain a practical understanding of how science communication works in a real-world context.

The effectiveness of these approaches hinges on understanding the audience's needs and backgrounds[9]. Tailoring science communication to the needs and backgrounds of the audience is a key aspect of effective science education, yet it's often overlooked. A scientific concept can be explained in many different ways, for instance, if you're discussing the immune system change with a group of fellow scientists, you might delve into the signalling pathways or the role of different cell types, but when explaining the same concept to a group of secondary school students or non-scientists, you'd need to simplify the language, use relatable analogies, and perhaps focus more on the relationship to disease and vaccination. Understanding your audience—their backgrounds, their level of knowledge, and their interests—is therefore critical. It can mean the difference between a clear, engaging explanation and a confusing, disengaging one. If your audience doesn't understands what you're saying, or if they find it irrelevant or uninteresting, you've lost them. To address this, we can incorporate exercises into the curriculum that emphasise audience-specific communication. For example, students could be tasked with explaining the same scientific concept to different audience groups. They might present to their peers, to younger students, or to a general audience. In each case, they would need to adjust their language, the complexity of their explanations, and the examples they use. Table 9.1 gives an example of tailoring communication to different audiences.

In each case, the underlying concept—the immune system—remains the same. However, the way you explain it changes significantly depending on the audience's background and understanding. This is where the skill of audience-specific communication comes into play. It's not just about knowing the science, but also knowing how to convey it in a way that resonates with different groups of people. Incorporating exercises in the curriculum that emphasise this skill can be tremendously beneficial. By practising explaining the same concept in different ways, students can gain a deeper understanding of the subject while also enhancing their communication skills. This, in turn, can help make science more accessible and engaging to a wider range of people.

It's not just the audience's needs and backgrounds that matter but also the platform on which the information is shared. If we stick with the immune system, when presenting this topic in a scientific journal or at a professional conference, the communication can be detailed and technical, complete with specialised terminology. These platforms cater to peers in the field who can

Table 9.1 Tailoring to different audiences

Audience	Tailoring
Biomedical science students/professionals	Intricacies of innate and adaptive immunity, the role of T-cells and B-cells, and the complex signalling pathways involved in an immune response. Might use specialised language, discuss recent research in the field, and possibly explore various immune diseases and their mechanisms.
Non-scientific audience	Here we can use analogies – we can liken the immune system to a body's defence force, fighting against harmful invaders such as viruses and bacteria. T-cells and B-cells could be described as specialised soldiers, each with their own unique strategies for combating these threats. And instead of going into detail about signalling pathways, we might focus on how vaccines help train this defence force to recognise and fight specific diseases.
Younger students	Here we would need to be even more simplified and engaging. We could use storytelling to make the concept more relatable, perhaps creating a narrative about the body being a castle, the pathogens being dragons, and the immune cells being knights defending the castle.

readily comprehend the jargon and complex concepts involved. If the same topic is being presented to a non-scientific audience through mass media or a public presentation, the strategy should shift towards clarity and simplicity. Terms like T-cells might be referred to as 'disease-fighting cells', and the immune response might be described as the body's way of 'fighting off harmful invaders'. The aim here is to deliver an understandable and relatable overview without overloading the audience with technical details. In a classroom setting, particularly with younger students, you could employ more engaging methods such as storytelling or gamification. Social media, on the other hand, offers a unique challenge due to its diverse audience and format constraints. Platforms like Twitter, with its character limit, necessitate a concise, punchy description of the immune system. On Instagram, which is more visual, you might share an engaging infographic or short animation showing how the immune system works.

These examples underscore the importance of flexibility and adaptability in science communication. The same core information can, and should, be presented differently based on the audience's knowledge level and the platform's specific context. Incorporating this understanding into the science curriculum can help students not only deepen their grasp of scientific concepts but also enhance their communication skills across various mediums. This adaptability is crucial for scientists and science communicators, making science more accessible and engaging for everyone.

The future of science communication education

As we move further into the digital age, the role of innovative communication channels in shaping the future of science communication becomes increasingly paramount. Social media, virtual reality, podcasts, blogs—these platforms are more than just mediums of expression[10]. They represent opportunities for scientists to reach broader audiences, to personalise complex ideas, and to foster engaging dialogues. A tweet about a breakthrough in gene therapy might inspire a young student to pursue a career in biomedical science. A podcast discussing the latest research on neurodegenerative diseases could offer hope to patients and their families. These cutting-edge platforms aren't just reshaping how scientific knowledge is transmitted; they're also redefining who gets to participate in the conversation. Traditionally, the realm of scientific discourse was largely confined to experts in the field—researchers, professors, and healthcare professionals. But in this digital era, that circle is expanding, individuals with an interest can now engage directly with scientific content tailored to their interests and level of understanding.

Consider the burgeoning trend of citizen science projects, these initiatives invite the general public to contribute to scientific research, be it through data collection, pattern recognition, or problem-solving. Projects like eBird[11] or Zooniverse[12] don't just benefit the scientific community through crowdsourcing; they also promote scientific literacy and foster a sense of investment in scientific discovery among participants. The impact of this democratisation of science communication is twofold. First, it facilitates a richer, more diverse dialogue around science. The inclusion of various perspectives can lead to fresh insights, nuanced discussions, and innovative solutions. Second, it empowers the public. When people are given the tools to engage with science—when they feel heard, involved, and informed—they're more likely to trust and support scientific endeavours. They can also become advocates for science in their own communities, further extending the reach of science communication. However, it's important to remember that with this expanded reach and participation comes an increased responsibility to communicate science accurately. Misunderstandings and misinformation can spread just as quickly as accurate information, if not more so. Therefore, honing the ability to communicate complex scientific ideas clearly in our students, without oversimplification or distortion, becomes increasingly important.

The issue of misinformation is an increasing concern in today's digitised society. The scientific community is not immune to this problem. In the vast expanse of the internet, flawed studies and sensationalised findings can easily take root, potentially leading the public down a path of misunderstanding and mistrust. In addressing this challenge, future curricula must prioritise critical thinking and information literacy alongside communication skills. This multifaceted approach is crucial to empowering students to tackle the spread of misinformation effectively. For instance, teaching students to identify and scrutinise sources can greatly help in distinguishing reliable information from the unreliable. Who conducted the study? Was it published in a peer-reviewed journal? Is the claim backed by evidence, or is it merely conjecture? These are essential questions that students must learn to ask when consuming scientific content. In tandem, students must also develop the ability to communicate their findings in a clear and responsible manner. This means avoiding hype, respecting the limitations of their studies, and framing their findings within the broader scientific context. By learning to translate their scientific insights into accessible language without compromising accuracy, students can contribute to a more informed and nuanced public discourse about science. It's also crucial to recognise the reciprocal relationship between communication and literacy skills. As students become better communicators, they're likely to develop a stronger understanding of the complexities and nuances of science, thus honing their information literacy. Similarly, as they enhance their critical thinking and evaluative skills, they can apply these insights to improve their own communication strategies.

Enhanced science communication education could precipitate profound changes in the field of biomedical science. Currently, the intricate details of biomedical research often remain confined within the walls of laboratories and academic journals. However, if these details were effectively communicated to diverse audiences, we could see a transformation in the public's understanding and engagement with biomedical science. Take, for example, the discussion around vaccines. Misunderstandings about vaccine development and safety have led to hesitation and outright refusal in some groups. Yet, if scientists could clearly articulate the rigorous testing procedures, the scientific consensus on vaccine safety, and the importance of herd immunity, we might witness an increased acceptance and a decrease in preventable diseases. Similarly, if we consider genetic modification, a topic often shrouded in controversy and misinformation, enhanced communication skills could facilitate a more informed dialogue, helping the public understand the potential benefits and risks rather than the discourse being driven by fear and misunderstanding. Instead, it could be guided by well-substantiated facts and a nuanced understanding of the science involved. Enhanced science communication could also influence policy-making[13]. Elected officials, informed by clear, accessible summaries of the latest research, could make decisions that better reflect scientific consensus. Policies on public health, environmental protection, and research funding could be more evidence-based, leading to improved outcomes.

The benefits of strong science communication skills extend beyond public understanding and can considerably improve interdisciplinary collaborations, accelerating innovation in the process[14]. For example, biomedical research generates enormous amounts of data—whether it's from genomics, proteomics, or metabolomics studies. To make sense of this data, scientists need sophisticated computational tools and algorithms. Here, computer scientists can lend their expertise, but this requires effective communication between the two fields. This isn't just about data handover; it's about clearly communicating the research question, explaining the nature of the data, and discussing the expected outcome. In return, the computer scientist shares their findings in a way that the biomedical researcher can understand and apply. Both parties must learn to speak a common language to bridge their knowledge gaps and work efficiently. Encouraging such interdisciplinary communication doesn't only benefit individual projects; it can foster a broader culture of collaboration. This breaks down the barriers between disciplines, leading to a more interconnected and dynamic scientific environment.

The imperative for integrating comprehensive science communication training into biomedical science courses is clear. It is a crucial thread that weaves through every aspect of a graduate's career path, societal engagement, interdisciplinary collaboration, and our collective responsibility to counter misinformation. Biomedical science, by its very nature, is complex and filled with intricate concepts that can seem incomprehensible to those outside the field. Yet, its implications extend far beyond lab walls, influencing public health policies, pharmaceutical advancements, and our understanding of human health and disease. The ability to break down this complexity, to transform the abstract and the arcane into narratives that captivate, educate, and inspire, is a skill that cannot be sidelined. As we prepare students to step into their roles as the next generation of researchers, educators, policy influencers, and scientific thought leaders, we have a responsibility to equip them with tools that will enable them to traverse the path successfully. The skill to communicate effectively—transcending jargon, tailoring messages for different audiences, and fostering an engaging dialogue around scientific issues—is one such tool.

Science communication serves as a bridge, connecting biomedical scientists with the public, policymakers, interdisciplinary collaborators, and even peers within their own field. Each audience requires a different approach, a different language, and a different level of detail. The ability to navigate these nuances, to shift between the complexities of a research paper and the simplicity required for a social media post, is a critical asset in today's digitised, interconnected world. In an era where misinformation can spread rapidly and create significant public health challenges, it's more important than ever for biomedical scientists to be active participants in the scientific dialogue. The ability to not only communicate accurate information but also debunk pseudoscience and misinformation is a key responsibility and can influence public opinion and policy decisions. By promoting science communication education, we equip students to succeed. Our students, well-versed in communication, could inspire the next generation and by bringing the excitement and importance of biomedical research to schools, media, and public forums, they could motivate more students to pursue careers in science.

Case study: Up-Goer Five Challenge

As part of our Science Communication module, one of the assessments is the production of a summary of a student's research project using both standard scientific language and in the format of the Up-Goer Five Challenge. Students also reflect on the differences between the two methods and how it has changed their perspective on talking about their project (Figure 9.1).

The Up Goer Five Challenge is a communication exercise that involves explaining complex or technical concepts using only the thousand most common words in the English (American) language. The name 'Up Goer Five' comes from the fact that the challenge was inspired by a diagram of a Saturn V rocket by Randall Munroe labelled using only such common words[15,16]. The challenge requires participants to simplify their language and avoid using jargon or technical terms, which can be especially challenging when explaining complex subjects like the research projects. It encourages creativity and forces students to think critically about how to convey their knowledge of their project in a clear and accessible way, using only simple language that can be easily understood by a wide audience.

At its core, the Up-Goer Five Challenge is an exercise in simplicity and clarity. Stripping scientific ideas down to their most fundamental components allows us to bypass the jargon that often alienates non-experts. By using language that is universally accessible, we ensure our message resonates with a broader audience. This approach cultivates an essential skill: the ability to demystify complex concepts, a cornerstone of effective science communication. It also promotes creative thinking—with a limited number of words available, students are encouraged to find innovative ways to express their

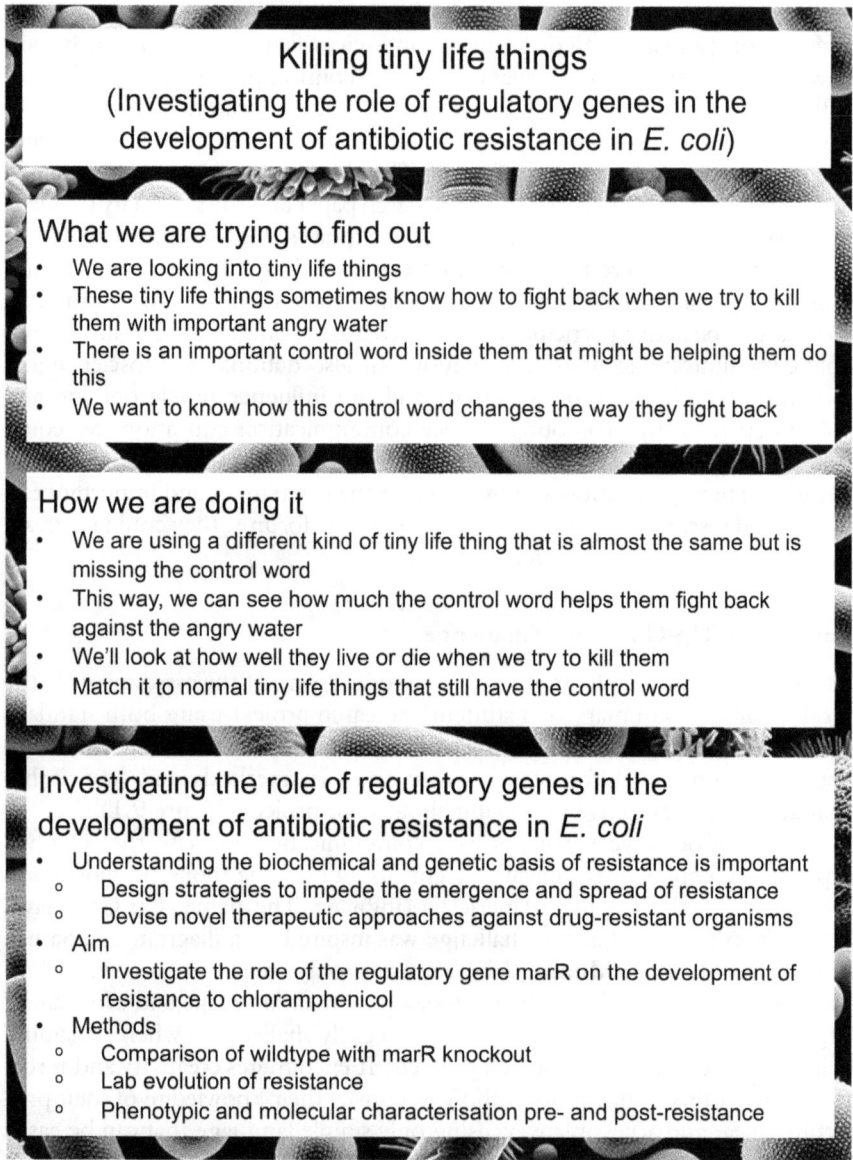

Killing tiny life things
(Investigating the role of regulatory genes in the development of antibiotic resistance in *E. coli*)

What we are trying to find out
- We are looking into tiny life things
- These tiny life things sometimes know how to fight back when we try to kill them with important angry water
- There is an important control word inside them that might be helping them do this
- We want to know how this control word changes the way they fight back

How we are doing it
- We are using a different kind of tiny life thing that is almost the same but is missing the control word
- This way, we can see how much the control word helps them fight back against the angry water
- We'll look at how well they live or die when we try to kill them
- Match it to normal tiny life things that still have the control word

Investigating the role of regulatory genes in the development of antibiotic resistance in *E. coli*
- Understanding the biochemical and genetic basis of resistance is important
  - Design strategies to impede the emergence and spread of resistance
  - Devise novel therapeutic approaches against drug-resistant organisms
- Aim
  - Investigate the role of the regulatory gene marR on the development of resistance to chloramphenicol
- Methods
  - Comparison of wildtype with marR knockout
  - Lab evolution of resistance
  - Phenotypic and molecular characterisation pre- and post-resistance

Figure 9.1 An example slide set.

thoughts. It's about finding new metaphors and crafting illustrative examples. In other words, it stimulates the development of storytelling techniques, another key aspect of compelling communication. One of the main benefits of this exercise is that it can deepen students' understanding of their projects. In attempting to simplify their language, they must engage deeply with the subject matter, distilling complex ideas to their core principles. This process not only reinforces their grasp of their understanding of their projects but can also shed new light on its nuances. This tool can be a stepping stone to more tailored communication approaches as well. Once students master the simple explanation, they can then learn to adjust the complexity of their language based on their audience's knowledge and background.

Typically, students find starting this assessment difficult, it can initially feel daunting. The task of distilling their understanding of their research project into only the most commonly used words in the English language can be intimidating, particularly if they feel they haven't yet solidified their understanding. The act of breaking down their project to its core elements is a crucial part of the assessment, but it is often where students struggle the most. They fear oversimplification and the loss of the nuances of their research or simply find it challenging to step back from the specialist terminology they're accustomed to. For students deeply engaged in their research project, it's easy to lose sight of the fact that what seems basic or obvious to them may not be to an outsider. This perspective shift—to view their work through the eyes of a layperson—can be a difficult adjustment. However, these initial difficulties are precisely why the Up-Goer Five challenge is such a valuable learning tool. It pushes students out of their comfort zones and forces them to approach their work from a new angle. It encourages them to delve deeper into their understanding of their project, as they must truly comprehend a concept to explain it simply.

Overall, the use of this challenge has a positive effect on students. They report talking more to non-expert family and friends about their projects and their language and through this process they come to better understand their projects and how to simplify these ideas. This is seen in the comments made by students as part of the reflection part of the assessment (Table 9.2). Students found the scientific language section easier but the simplified section helped them to develop confidence in their knowledge and their understanding of the role of language in science communication.

Table 9.2 Student comments from their reflections

This assessment shows not only the importance of making science accessible for all but the content relevant and engaging for the target group where use of language plays an important role.

Audience has to be fully engaged where the point of this exercise was to appreciate the need to make science accessible for all.

It helped me understand that there are other words that can be used just as effectively.

Made me realise how far my scientific knowledge and vocabulary has improved over the past couple of years.

Enjoyed having to think around the subject and come up with different ways of portraying information.

Help bridge the gap between the scientific community and the general public.

Making science more accessible for everyone.

Being able to express information in different ways, is a good skill to have as its application can be used in multiple situations.

Incorporating such exercises into the curriculum can be a powerful way to improve science communication skills. Students learn to adjust their language and presentation based on their audience, making their explanations more accessible and engaging. It's a vital skill for any scientist or science communicator, and one that our education system should strive to nurture more effectively.

Conclusion

The role of effective communication in biomedical science extends far beyond the confines of academia to encompass public engagement, policy influence, and interdisciplinary collaboration. The ability to translate complex scientific concepts into clear, accessible narratives is not just a valuable skill; it's an essential tool in the modern biomedical scientist's repertoire. This importance is magnified in an era where misinformation can rapidly propagate, necessitating a concerted effort to develop both scientific literacy and communication proficiency within the educational framework.

The integration of science communication into the curricula is crucial is important to support the development of a new generation of scientists who are not only adept in their technical fields but also skilled communicators. This skill set is vital for bridging the gap between the scientific community and the general public, policymakers, and professionals from other disciplines. Effective communication promotes a deeper understanding of biomedical science, encouraging a scientifically literate society that appreciates the value of research and evidence-based decision-making. It also enhances the employability of graduates, opening doors to a diverse range of career opportunities where the ability to articulate scientific knowledge is highly valued.

The challenges posed by the digital age, particularly the proliferation of misinformation, further underscore the need for robust science communication education. As the landscape of information dissemination evolves, so too must the strategies employed to engage with it. Biomedical science education must adapt, prioritising the development of critical evaluation skills alongside communication proficiency. This dual approach is key for empowering students to navigate the complex web of information that characterises the digital era, enabling them to discern credible sources and combat the spread of pseudoscience.

Looking ahead, the future of science communication in biomedical science education is poised for transformative growth. The expanding role of digital platforms presents both challenges and opportunities for science communicators. The ability to navigate these platforms effectively and adapting the message to the medium and audience, will be a key skill for future scientists. In this context, the focus on communication skills in biomedical science curricula is more than just a necessity; it's an opportunity to shape a more informed, engaged, and scientifically literate society. By equipping students with the tools to communicate science effectively, we empower them to play a crucial role in shaping public discourse, influencing policy, and driving scientific innovation.

References

1. Brownell SE, Price JV, Steinman L. Science communication to the general public: Why we need to teach undergraduate and graduate students this skill as part of their formal scientific training. *J Undergrad Neurosci Educ.* 2013;12(1):E6–E10.
2. Bucchi M Facing the challenges of science communication 2.0: Quality, credibility and expertise. *EFSA J.* 2019;17(Suppl 1):e170702.
3. Mercer-Mapstone L, Kuchel L. Teaching Scientists to Communicate: Evidence-based assessment for undergraduate science education. *Int J Sci Educ.* 2015;37(10):1613–1638.
4. Muhammed TS, Mathew SK. The disaster of misinformation: A review of research in social media. *Int J Data Sci Anal.* 2022;13(4):271–285.
5. Howell EL, Brossard D. (Mis)informed about what? What it means to be a science-literate citizen in a digital world. *Proc Natl Acad Sci U S A.* 2021;118(15). doi:10.1073/pnas.1912436117
6. Gade S, Chari S. Case-based learning in endocrine physiology: An approach toward self-directed learning and the development of soft skills in medical students. *Adv Physiol Educ.* 2013;37(4):356–360.
7. Dewi H Project based learning techniques to improve speaking skills. *Engl Educ J.* 2016;7(3):341–359.
8. Kokotsaki D, Menzies V, Wiggins A. Project-based learning: A review of the literature. *Improv Sch.* 2016;19(3):267–277.
9. Fischhoff B The sciences of science communication. *Proc Natl Acad Sci U S A.* 2013;110 Suppl 3:14033–14039.
10. Gergő PD. Various challenges of science communication in teaching generation Z: An urgent need for paradigm shift and embracing digital learning. *OpEE.* 2016;3(6). doi:10.3311/ope.146
11. eBird – Discover a new world of birding. Accessed July 3, 2023. https://ebird.org/home
12. Zooniverse. Accessed July 3, 2023. https://www.zooniverse.org/
13. Pulido-Salgado M, Castaneda Mena FA. Bringing policymakers to science through communication: A perspective from Latin America. *Front Res Metr Anal.* 2021;6:654191.
14. Kahlor L, Stout P. *Understanding and Communicating Science: New Agendas in Communication.* Routledge; 2009.
15. Rowan C Science in ten hundred words: The 'up-goer five' challenge. *Sci Am.* https://blogs.scientificamerican.com/guest-blog/science-in-ten-hundred-words-the-up-goer-five-challenge/
16. Munroe R Up Goer Five. xkcd. Accessed July 3, 2023. https://xkcd.com/1133/

10 The value of Scicomm from the students' perspective

Building identity and professional values

Sara Smith and Martin P Khechara

The higher education landscape

The Dearing Review, which called for widening participation and greater student diversity across the Higher Education (HE) sector is now over 25 years old[1]. In the intervening years educational reform along with labour market changes have contributed to a rapidly changing landscape for HE. The Office for Students (OfS)[2] came into force at the start of 2018 with the role of holding universities to account and to promote students' interests. Their regulatory framework aims to ensure the provision of a high-quality academic experience for all students, enabling them to progress into employment or further study with qualifications that 'hold their value over time'[2]. Meeting these challenges of contemporary society has resulted in a move within HE to ensure that degrees are more applicable to the world of work[3], providing students with the opportunity to develop the essential skills to practice in their chosen field. Education and training have been reconceptualised through human capital theory as principally economic approaches and essential to participation in the global economy. Graduate attributes are defined as the attributes, competencies, and insights that a university collectively believes its students should ideally cultivate during their academic journey to fundamentally influence the impact these individuals can subsequently have in their chosen careers and as members of society[4].

The concept of capability emerged from the UK in the mid-1980s as the need for a more competitive workforce, able to adapt to rapid changes, was acknowledged[5]. The ensuing changes seen in approaches to supporting learning and guidance within government directives are anchored firmly in the neoliberal policy-making agenda of the Labour Party during the 1990s and as a response to globalisation[6]. The objective of the capability movement was to break down the dichotomy between training and education by embracing the perceptions of education and training within a practical approach to learning that addressed the wider picture[7]. Capability is seen as an essential learning outcome that supports individuals to integrate enquiry and evidence into practice enhancement and professional learning[8]. The concept of capability draws on the work of Schön[9], and what he referred to as 'professional artistry';

DOI: 10.4324/9781003383994-15

preparing students to apply their knowledge in unfamiliar settings. Capability entails individuals bringing together their knowledge and skills, including personal attributes, to effectively respond to and tackle a range of circumstances, both known and unknown[10]. A capable individual is one who not only has the required knowledge and skills for a role but also has the confidence to apply these in varied and challenging situations, whilst continuing to develop their specialist skills and knowledge[7]. The ability of individuals to adopt this approach to practice is essential for complex and rapidly changing environments such as the healthcare setting.

Astin's student development theory[11] highlights how the experiences of students during their time in HE impact their learning. He theorised that the greater the student's involvement in their studies, the greater the student's learning and personal development. Increasingly, HE is discussed in terms of its contribution to human capital, an individual's employability and to economic growth. As a result of this focus, student experience and graduate outcomes are often evaluated against these metrics. However, research suggests that a 'gap' exists between what are articulated as graduate attributes and the reality of the student learning experience[12]. Graduate attributes are often reduced to generic skills and linked to the learning outcomes of specific modules rather than being clearly grounded in the authentic application of learning.

Crossling, Heagney, and Thomas[13] underline how fostering students' engagement in their studies and university life is a fundamental strategy for improving student retention, success, and outcomes. A student-responsive curriculum where students are immersed in authentic curriculum content and tasks that are challenging and relevant to their lives and futures is recognised as invaluable in promoting student engagement, success in their studies, and the development of capability for practice.

Adopting student-centred learning approaches enables students to play a more active role in their learning processes. Rather than the didactic large lecture format, active learning embraces experiential, problem-based and project-based learning where students and tutors work collaboratively. Pedagogies that engage students as active learners, rather than passive individuals who receive knowledge, acknowledge students' views and experiences and enable them to engage and contribute to the conversations. Many students still experience university life as isolated learners, disconnected from the learning of others. Tinto[14] identified that students not only benefit from being part of 'learning communities' but also enjoy the experience. He suggests that being part of such a learning community shapes interactions between students and facilitates their learning not only within the classroom setting but also their wider community[14]. Such an approach develops a student's capability for practice. It allows the student to evolve, recognising the scope of their intended profession, and enables ongoing development and progression of skills into more advanced and refined practice[15,16].

The challenge for academics is to foster this learning environment enabling students to move from the periphery to core membership of the community[17] and so develop the skills required to be a capable individual. This chapter evaluates the potential role of science communication (Scicomm) through community engagement activities to develop a pedagogical approach that supports the development of the capability of individuals grounded within authentic learning experiences.

What is science communication?

Scicomm is a rapidly growing area of practice and research that aims to educate, entertain, and engage the public with and about science, with engagement being the overriding priority. A vast range of approaches to achieving these goals exist including traditional journalism with magazine articles, television and radio shows, live or face-to-face events such as public lectures or science busking, and online interactions including blogs, social media, and Citizen Science[18]. Each adopts a dialogic model of engaging the public with science to support effective and meaningful communication and outreach. The communicators (Scicommers) delivering the engagement events and the public attending these events both benefit when communication is genuine and grounded in good public engagement practice[19]. Scicomm often focuses upon researchers or other engagement practitioners delivering sessions to communicate research or scientific topics of interest to the public, raising awareness and supporting greater understanding around specific issues. For the scientists involved this provides them with essential personal development opportunities. Research into the benefits of participating in Scicomm events has mainly focused upon post-graduate and doctoral students with limited studies addressing the benefit of incorporating Scicomm into an undergraduate science curriculum. Extant studies that do focus on undergraduate students merely concentrate on the students' perceptions of Scicomm skills and the lack of coherent opportunities for students to learn and develop these skills across year levels[20].

What is student community engagement?

Undergraduate student engagement in community-based projects has been shown to support the development of graduate attributes – providing real-life experiences to support the development of the skills required for future employment[21]. Student community engagement (SCE) in the context of this study is defined as both off-site and on-site activities by students with the community with the intention of conveying a benefit to the public. This approach draws upon Battistoni's concept of Service Learning which offered a model that integrates 'liberal teaching, experiential learning, critical reflection, community service and citizen education into a pedagogy of freedom'[22]. Students often struggle to understand the relevance of their studies to real-world situations or future careers and also have a limited understanding of community issues or the barriers others may face. Engagement in meaningful activities ensures greater authenticity of experience for students[23].

Case studies: Student community engagement

In order to redress the limited opportunity afforded to students to engage in authentic application of learning by providing them with the chance of designing, developing and delivering community outreach activities we developed an opportunity for student-community engagement. The aim was to develop learner's Scicomm skills through engaging with the public. In presenting students with this opportunity, we evaluated whether by involving undergraduate students in outreach activities and developing their Scicomm skills we could deliver on Astin's development theory[11], and provide an authentic learning experience to promote the development of capability and essential graduate attributes, helping students to move from the periphery into core membership of their learning community.

Biomedical scientists (BMSs) carry out a range of laboratory and scientific tests that are essential in supporting the diagnosis, treatment and development of patients. Success in modern healthcare relies on the accuracy and efficiency of work by BMSs since patients' lives and the treatment of illness depend on their skill and knowledge[24]. Tutors on the undergraduate course for BMSs are tasked with supporting the students to relate their academic studies to the world of work and to gain the skills and knowledge required to become an effective member of the workplace community.

We employed a case study approach to explore the role of Scicomm in supporting students during their academic journey. Yin[25] defines case studies as allowing researchers to explain, describe, or explore events or phenomena in the everyday contexts in which they occur. He categorises case studies as explanatory, exploratory, or descriptive. An exploratory case study approach enables not only the

> 'what' but also the 'how' and 'why' questions to be answered while taking into consideration how a phenomenon is affected by the context within which it is situated[26]. An exploratory case study approach is, therefore, valuable in developing an understanding of the impact of *'being a Scicommer'*

on biomedical science students, whether it influences their perception of their studies, in what way, how and why? In this study we have taken an interpretivist epistemological stance to allow us to understand the individual and shared social meanings of community engagement through Scicomm. A broad research question was posed: What impact does becoming a 'Scicommer' have on undergraduate biomedical science students' university experience?

Case study 1 – Developing an informal science event

A group of final-year undergraduate biomedical science students (n = 4) developed and delivered an informal science event at a local college for students currently studying post-16 science pathways. The activity formed their honours research project and required them to answer the research question – *What impact does informal science learning have on college students' perceptions of the field of biomedical science?* Each student was tasked with developing an interactive 'playground' activity that demonstrated a specific discipline within the field of biomedical science to support the college students to develop a deeper understanding of the importance of this field of healthcare science and its relevance to them as individuals. An action research approach was adopted by the students starting with them firstly visiting a pathology laboratory to develop their own understanding of the daily work of a BMS. Based upon their visits, the students then designed an interactive activity for college students that would provide them with a deeper understanding of the roles and responsibilities of BMSs and how their essential day-to-day practice impacts their own lives. Finally, the students evaluated the impact of their informal science learning activities via questionnaires. The honours project module is assessed through a dissertation and poster presentation. As part of their standard dissertation report students were also asked to write a reflective account addressing the experience of being involved in a community engagement event as a science communicator from the initial conception to delivery of their activities. This did not form part of the students' assessment for the module and limited guidance for the reflective report was provided. They were asked to talk about their own personal journey and reflect upon what the experience meant to them.

Case study 2 – Delivery of Scicomm activities

Case study 2 involved students delivering Scicomm activities as volunteers and separate to their formal studies (n = 4). Students were involved in the delivery of activities as part of a wider science festival held at the university. The festival ran over two days. The first day was for primary schools and focused upon engaging children in activities related to science, technology, engineering, and maths (STEM) to ignite their interest and encourage greater participation in these subject areas. The second day was open to the public and the wider community. The biomedical science students collaborated with academic staff to design and deliver activities on both days. Guests were able to take part in the activities as they wandered around the festival. Each activity had a theme and was designed to raise the children's and publics' awareness of the roles of BMSs in the workplace and the skills and knowledge required for the profession. Students did not have to design the workshops but were expected to develop and personalise them, making sure that they were fun and informative for all age groups.

Focus groups were held with the four students three weeks after the event. The focus groups began with set questions posed around how students felt about being involved in the festival and what they enjoyed most. However, since the value of focus groups is that they allow rich data to be elicited from the interactivity of group members[27] students were encouraged to lead the discussions to allow perceptions and interpretations to be challenged and uncovered. A deliberative approach[28] enables a socially constructed view of experiences, allowing individuals to react to and build upon the focus group discussions. Each focus group was recorded and transcripts were made of the recordings.

Student reflective reports and focus group transcripts were anonymised and analysed using thematic analysis. below.

We used open coding which allowed codes to be developed describing, naming or classifying concepts through the use of simple words or a short sequence of words. Analysis of the codes allowed the identification of key themes within the data to address the research question.

Table 10.1 provides an example of the development of initial and focused codes from reflective reports and focus group transcripts.

Findings

Students involved in both case studies were extremely enthusiastic about being involved in the study and their role within the community engagement events. As outlined, analysis of the reflective reports and transcripts provided a range of codes. Clustering of codes provided three key categories: emotional, cognitive and behavioural aspects of the students' experiences. These are summarised in Figure 10.1. In developing and analysing these three categories the

Table 10.1 Example of initial and focused coding of reflective reports and focus group transcripts

Reflective account excerpts (initial coding)	*Focused codes*
I realised that I was good at talking to people....you could say that the project [delivering scicomm activity] changed my opinion of my own skills	Metacognition Self-efficacy
These experiences [delivering informal science activities] moulded myself into a more rounded individual	Personal Development
The journey of creating ideas and working with fellow colleagues was exciting...inventing the intervention was very exciting	Motivating Collegiality Autonomy
Transcript excerpts – initial coding	**Focused codes**
I developed being able to speak to people. In a degree that is something that doesn't really get addressed	Confidence Relationships Personal development
For me it was the transfer of skills [delivering the workshops]. If you can do something in a situation it can help you do something in another situation	Metacognition Personal development
It was like you belong to the university, you are part of the faculty, it's not just about knowing things	Identity Relationships

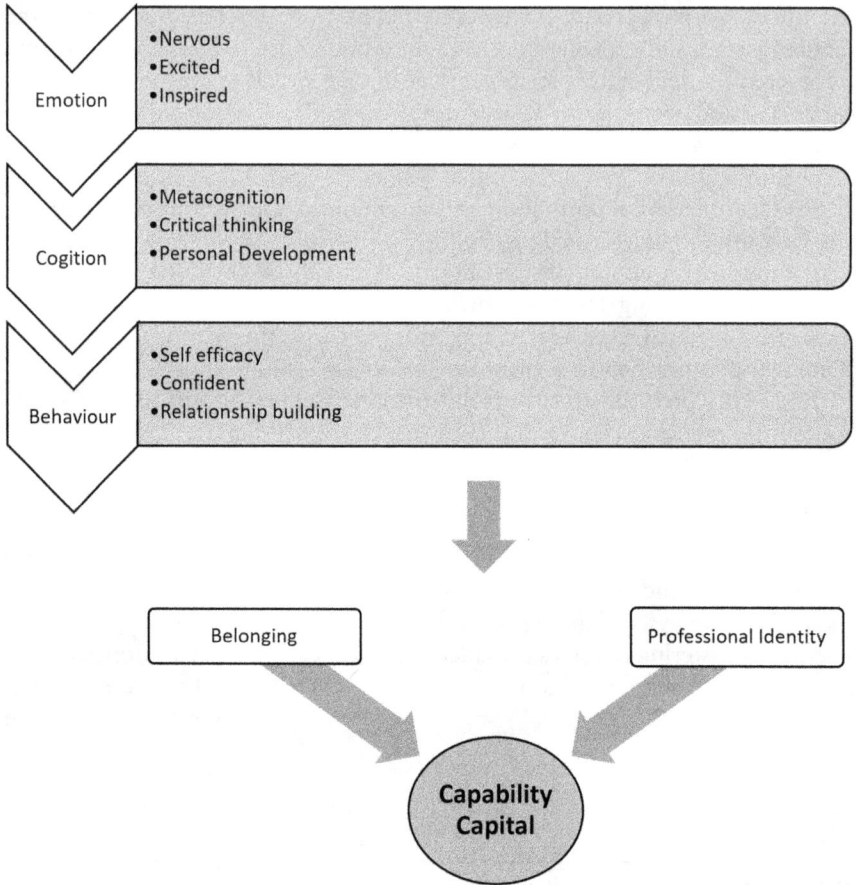

Figure 10.1 Clustering of focused codes to show the development of three categories and two key themes of belonging and professional identity fostering the development of 'capability capital'.

themes of belonging and professionalism were identified to support a substantive theory of the role of Scicomm in fostering what we refer to as 'capability capital' within the undergraduate students involved.

Emotions

A range of different emotions were evoked in the students in both case studies. Students identified feelings of being both scared as well as excited about their involvement in the events. However, the experience did not equate to negative emotions and even the nervous feelings were identified as resulting in a positive outcome and something they had not previously experienced in their studies:

The journey for me was very nerve racking, I knew though that informal science learning is a very effective method, this excited me to be involved.....to eventually spark an interest in participants to be involved in science.

(CS1-1)

Prior to the activity I was very apprehensive, I was anxious about my activity... once students came flowing in it became easier...it inspired me.

(CS1-2)

The excerpts from students' reflective accounts identify that although initially being involved in Scicomm moved students outside of their comfort zone in both case studies the act of being involved and supporting others to develop a passion for science was perceived as exciting and something positive to be part of. As the students started to see the children and young adults enjoying the activities and demonstrating a genuine interest, they themselves were inspired.

In case study 1 the feeling of inspiration that the students reported resulted in motivation and greater engagement within their studies. Students took ownership of their own learning since they could see the positive impact that their activities were having on the children. This inspiration and motivation fostered greater involvement in the subject area of biomedical science resulting in them acknowledging the development of a deeper grasp of subject knowledge:

[developing and delivering the interventions] *helped me effectively understand my own field strongly as well.*

(CS1-1)

This reflects Jung's work[23] highlighting how engagement in meaningful activities ensures greater authenticity of experience for students. By sharing their knowledge of biomedical science with others the students in both case studies were involved in 'authentic experiences' that gave currency to their learning and in turn stimulated cognitive changes. For the students in case study 2, the initial nervousness acknowledged as a result of running activities for children and not knowing how to react to questions was also replaced by enjoyment and motivation. Students commented that it was '*definitely a positive experience*' (CS2-1) and that it made them '*feel a bit more productive*' (CS2-1). This would suggest that students felt that being involved in Scicomm gave them a greater feeling of achievement during their university journey not previously afforded by their studies.

Cognitive

Engaging students as active learners, rather than as passive individuals who receive knowledge is known to support a deeper approach to learning and to strengthen their understanding of a topic area[29]. In both case studies students were very vocal about how involvement in Scicomm had impacted their learning and their ability to articulate their knowledge to others. Coding identified how students acknowledged that developing and delivering interventions improved their subject knowledge and understanding. It was even credited to supporting the development of a more critical approach:

> [Scicomm intervention] *has helped to enhance my scientific writing skills and develop critical thinking when I look at my previous studies.*
>
> (CS1-2)

This student was inspired by being involved in Scicomm which in turn motivated and engaged them as an active learner within their studies. The result was that they took ownership of their learning and not only developed a deeper understanding of their subject but importantly, started to acknowledge and develop many of the essential graduate attributes that are so difficult to foster by traditional approaches to curriculum delivery alone.

Students highlighted how delivering informal science sessions provided them with a greater awareness of their own understanding and abilities. When talking about being involved in the science festival one of the students in case study 2 commented that:

> I was quite conscious that I'm still a student...but I do know something and I do have some knowledge too.
>
> (CS2-1)

Scicomm supported a metacognitive shift within the students involved:

> I think it kind of solidified my ground really, made me realise what I was doing, 'I'm actually doing biomed here!'... this is actually my area and I was kind of solidifying the fact.
>
> (CS2-3)

The excerpt shows how by being immersed in their field of study and applying their knowledge to practice students started to recognise their own abilities and to make the links between concepts they were learning and how they relate to practice *'solidifying facts' (CS2-3)*.

In addition, the students acknowledged how they developed the ability to think on their feet and make decisions about what to do next or how to develop their session:

> There was a couple of children that came with their parents who were home schooled.... they had more special needs.... so we engaged with them more.... made sure they knew what was going on.
>
> (CS2-4)

Students in both case studies were seen to adapt and develop their approach, decision making without requesting additional support, developing greater independence which in turn also led to greater confidence in their own ability.

In both case studies, 'development as a person' was recognised by all of the students involved. Each of the students felt that 'becoming a Scicommmer' had fostered their personal development as well as impacting on their scientific knowledge and skills.

> I developed being able to speak to people. In a degree that is something that doesn't really get addressed.
>
> (CS1-3)

This final-year student acknowledged that they would not previously have just chatted to others, even to tutors and peers whom they were already familiar with. Another student suggested that they now felt a more rounded individual as a result of the experience:

> These experiences [delivering informal science activities] moulded myself into a more rounded individual.
>
> (CS1-4)

This suggests that they identified that being involved in Scicomm provided learning and development not already afforded within their current studies. Development of self consequently led to a greater ability to interact with peers and colleagues. In turn this was seen to make students feel more comfortable at university:

> [Talking about university life and interactions with tutors] *It has made me feel more comfortable.*
>
> (CS2-4)

Linking into the emotional and cognitive shifts, students acknowledged how this initiated behavioural changes.

Behavioural

Each of the students highlighted how their confidence in both their knowledge and abilities grew as they took part in the events. An increase in their confidence was seen to foster greater communication skills, self-efficacy, perceptions of identity and relationship building.

One of the most marked changes that all students highlighted was the development of their confidence to communicate with others and at all levels. Students commented on this by saying:

My communication skills developed drastically....I had to communicate with teaching professionals' (CS1-2) and 'I realised that I was good at talking to people.

(CS1-3)

This emphasised how students acknowledged a change in their own behaviour and their ability to interact not just with the children but also with individuals in positions of authority.

Transcripts from case study 2 revealed that the students perceived a traditional degree as not supporting such behavioural changes:

[Discussing being involved in the event] "*It's developing being able to speak to people. In a degree that is something that doesn't really get addressed, I think obviously, moving forward we are going to have to be able to do that*".

(CS2-1)

Students' comments demonstrated that they are aware of the skills that they will need when they enter the workplace and appreciated that Scicomm did not just support them to develop and apply their subject-specific knowledge, but also to nurture generic graduate attributes. In acknowledging that they were developing a range of additional skills students' feeling of self-efficacy emerged within both case studies:

They actually wanted to know stuff [children]. There was none of 'er, what is she actually talking about' and they was interested. So I could get down on their level - I was more confident in talking to them towards the end of the day.

(CS2-3)

Bandura[30] named four sources of efficacy beliefs: mastery experiences, vicarious experiences, verbal persuasion, and emotional and physiological states. Each of these areas is addressed by 'being a Scicommmer'. Students in case study 1 acknowledged how mastering a task developed their self-efficacy:

After interacting with an item which I meticulously designed [informal science intervention] I began to see a more comfortable individual [children and young adults] who now understood the meaning of biomedical science and biochemistry. This increased my self-assurance.......it had a positive impact on me as the educator and the learner.

(CS1-4)

In designing and delivering a workshop for groups of children and young adults, students built their self-belief. They started to develop a resilient sense of self-efficacy since they had overcome obstacles, such as nerves and lack of confidence, through their effort and perseverance with their interventions.

In case study 2, the students experienced controlling the environment. They were required to manage the stalls that they ran and again, to overcome their initial unease:

> With the younger kids I had to calm myself down completely, get to their level, watch what I was saying, and change the language as well. The way I was talking to them, and my tone of voice..... after speaking to little kids, my confidence was a lot more.
>
> (CS2-4)

The opportunity to independently design and deliver an informal science intervention nurtured students' mastery of the task. When discussing what it was about the experience that supported their confidence in their own ability a student commented:

> I think it is about control and experience.
>
> (CS2-1)

However, in both case studies the students were also working as a team supporting and encouraging each other. Bandura[30] highlights vicarious experiences as important in the development of self-efficacy. Seeing people similar to ourselves succeed raises our beliefs that we too have the capabilities to master the activities needed for success in that area. This was clearly articulated by one of the students from case study 1:

> The journey of creating these ideas and working with fellow colleagues was exciting...working with fellow colleagues beside me motivating each other gave us the drive.
>
> (CS1-1)

As well as the positive impact of working alongside peers, students identified that they valued highly the relationships that they built with those that they saw as being in authority and representing the wider university community and said:

> Working with people like yourselves, and more senior people in the uni that kind of helped out a lot 'cus you are getting more of a chance to interact with them on a different level not just inside a lecture, and this does make you feel more comfortable 'cus you can see that they are people and you can approach them outside of lectures and that.
>
> (CS2-3)

Working alongside individuals who are seen as authority figures or specialists is seen to strengthen the students' belief in their own legitimacy within the university environment and confidence to join the 'community of practice'[17].

As students started to build relationships and become more confident individuals, they started to view themselves as positioned within the wider university community and adopted a stronger identity for themselves. In both case studies the language used by students demonstrated that they saw themselves more as BMSs rather than students studying biomedical science; building an identity. These feelings of belonging within the university community were expressed differently by the students in the two case studies. For the students in case study 1, 'being a Scicommmer' and developing their own intervention appeared to provide them with greater legitimacy as a scientist and this then strengthened their feelings of being part of the university community:

> My level of professional competency increased as I represented the University.
>
> (CS1-2)

Students used terms such as '*we as biomedical scientists*' (CS1-4) when referring to themselves and acknowledged increased feelings of identity as a scientist or practitioner which in turn provided a greater feeling of belonging. In contrast, the students in case study 2 focused more on how being involved in activities alongside the wider university community nurtured feelings of belonging.

> It was like you belong to the university, you are part of the faculty, it's not just about knowing things...you feel a bit more involved, you feel like, oh yeah, I know who I can go and talk to.
>
> (CS2-3)

The excerpt above highlights how working alongside tutors and other members of the university provided them with a feeling of permission to engage with this community. The feeling of belonging has been shown to be a critical factor in determining student retention[31] as well as nurturing student progression and achievement[32]. Identity development is an important part of preparation and training for a career and supports the student in moving from peripheral participation to full participation within the community of practice[17]. In both case studies, the development of a professional identity by the students was seen as providing them with a bridge across from the periphery of the community. Constructivist and sociocultural theories of learning emphasise the need for environments that encourage students to question and learn via active involvement which in turn supports the development of student capability[33]. Learning as an 'active person' through social engagement results in a different outcome to learning as an 'individual person'. It supports the construction of knowledge and understanding by drawing on others and through interactions with the environment, 'priority, perspective and value are continuously and inescapably generated in activity'[34].

The interactions and intersection of the categories of emotion, cognition and behaviour provided us with the two themes of belonging and professional identity. In fostering an environment where students perceived themselves as members of a group and started to build an identity within that community, individuals were seen to integrate enquiry and evidence into practice enhancement and professional learning[35]. Not only did they develop greater skills to deliver the Scicomm activity in a more confident and knowledgeable way, they also applied this approach to their wider subject area and grew in confidence within their own community of practice. Students were seen to evolve and acquire a deeper appreciation of the scope of their intended profession[36]. Initial findings suggest that developing capability or what we have called here 'capability capital' provides a way of describing and conceptualising how 'becoming a Scicommmer' affords students this 'entry ticket'. Evaluation of students' comments characterises 'capability capital' as an enabler, allowing students to see themselves as legitimate members of the university community, making a valuable and recognisable contribution. This in turn provides the student with greater personal and professional identity, delivering on Astin's development theory that the greater the student's involvement in their studies, the greater the student's learning and their personal development[37].

Our initial aim in involving students in Scicomm through community engagement was to evaluate whether it was able to support the development of some of the essential employability skills that are valued by employers but often a challenge to address within the standard curriculum. It is clear from the results of this study that involvement in Scicomm interventions is a powerful experiential way of engendering better communication skills, adaptability and resilience while providing a greater sense of professional identity and belonging. The emotionally transactional relationship developed during the action of communication within Scicomm allows the realisation that students are the experts and that they have an identity within their subject area and have become practitioners in their own right. Scicomm remains a highly effective tool to give employability-relevant graduate attributes that cannot be taught within the confines of a normal HE teaching programme. Further evaluation should be carried out to investigate the effectiveness of this form of communication for personal development with the aim to create work-ready socially efficacious graduates with increased capability capital.

Conclusion

The landscape of HE, particularly in biomedical science, has undergone significant transformation over the past decades, marked by an increasing emphasis on developing capabilities that extend beyond traditional academic skills. The shift towards embedding capabilities such as adaptability, effective communication, and a strong sense of professional identity in students reflects a response to the dynamic and complex nature of contemporary societal and professional environments. The integration of Scicomm and community engagement in the curriculum represents a strategic approach to cultivating these capabilities. These initiatives not only enhance students' understanding of their field but also develop essential soft skills like public engagement, adaptability, and the ability to translate complex scientific knowledge into accessible language. This approach is critical in preparing students to become competent professionals who can navigate and contribute to diverse settings, from academic research to public policy and healthcare delivery.

This shift in HE is also a response to the changing nature of the job market, where interdisciplinary skills and the ability to communicate across various platforms are increasingly valued. The case studies in this chapter highlight how these innovative teaching methods contribute to students' overall development. By engaging in these activities, students transition from being passive recipients of knowledge to becoming active participants in their learning community, gaining a sense of belonging and professional identity that is crucial for their future roles as biomedical professionals. These educational approaches also address the gap between the acquisition of theoretical knowledge and its practical, real-world application. The hands-on experience gained through Scicomm and community projects enhances students' employability and readiness to face the challenges and opportunities of their future careers.

Biomedical science education is increasingly focused on producing well-rounded, capable, and adaptable graduates. This holistic educational approach is instrumental in preparing students not only as professionals in their field but also as informed, communicative, and adaptable individuals who can effectively contribute to the broader society. This evolution in HE reflects a commitment to nurturing graduates who are equipped to navigate the complexities of a rapidly changing world, both professionally and socially.

References

1. Dearing, R Higher Education in the Learning Society: The National Committee of Enquiry into Higher Education. 1997. Published online 1997.
2. Office for Students. Home - Office for Students. Published online January 12, 2018. Accessed September 25, 2023. https://www.officeforstudents.org.uk/
3. Helyer R Aligning higher education with the world of work. *Higher Education, Skills and Work-Based Learning.* 2011;1(2):95–105.
4. Australian Technology Network. *Generic Capabilities of ATN University Graduates.* Teaching and Learning Committee, Australian Technology Network; 2000.
5. Hase S, Davis L. From competence to capability: The implications for human resource development and management. In: *Millennial Challenges in Management, Cybertechnology, and Leadership Education: Association of International Management, 17th Annual Conference.*; 1999. https://researchportal.scu.edu.au/esploro/fulltext/conferencePresentation/From-competence-to-capability-the-implications/991012820941902368?repId=1266995440002368&mId=1367476780002368&institution=61SCU_INST

6. Olssen M, Peters MA. Neoliberalism, higher education and the knowledge economy: From the free market to knowledge capitalism. *Journal of Education Policy.* 2005;20(3):313–345.

7. Stephenson J Capability and competence: Are they the same and does it matter? *Capability.* Published online 1994.

8. Zaikowski LA, Garrett JM. A three-tiered approach to enhance undergraduate education in bioethics. *Bioscience.* 2004;54(10):942–949.

9. Schön D Chapter 13: The crisis of professional knowledge and the pursuit of an epistemology of practice. *Counterpoints.* 2001;166:183–207.

10. Carryer J, Gardner G, Dunn S, Gardner A. The core role of the nurse practitioner: Practice, professionalism and clinical leadership. *Journal of Clinical Nursing.* 2007;16(10):1818–1825.

11. Astin AW. Student involvement: A developmental theory for higher education. In: *College Student Development and Academic Life.* Routledge; 2014:251–262.

12. Hughes C, Barrie S. Influences on the assessment of graduate attributes in higher education. *Assessment & Evaluation in Higher Education.* 2010;35(3):325–334.

13. Crossling G, Heagney M, Thomas L. Improving student retention in higher education. *Australian Higher Education Review.* Published online 2008.

14. Tinto V Learning better together: The impact of learning communities on student success. *Higher Education Monograph Series.* 2003;1(8):1–8

15. Kenyon C, Hase S. Moving from andragogy to heutagogy in vocational education. Published online 2001.

16. Smith S, Braszkiewicz W, Goncalves Barbosa Neto C, Mohammed B, McCulla D, Khechara M. Acknowledging the value of friendships and relationships in supporting personal and professional development. *Practice.* 2022;4(2):110–124.

17. Wenger E. Communities of practice: Learning, meaning, and identity. https://psycnet.apa.orgrecord. 1998;318. doi:10.1017/CBO9780511803932

18. Bultitude K The why and how of science communication. In: Rosulek P, ed. *Science Communication.* European Commission; 2011.

19. Clarke AE. A social worlds research adventure. In: Strauss A & Corbin J, ed. *Grounded Theory in Practice.* SAGE Publications Inc; 1997:63–94.

20. Mercer-Mapstone LD, Matthews KE. Student perceptions of communication skills in undergraduate science at an Australian research-intensive university. *Assessment & Evaluation in Higher Education.* 2017;42(1):98–114.

21. Knight-McKenna M, Felten P, Darby A. Student engagement with community. *New Directions for Teaching and Learning.* 2018;2018(154):65–74.

22. Battistoni R. Service learning, diversity, and the liberal arts curriculum. *Liberal Education.* Published online 1995:30.

23. Jung J Assessing learning from a student community engagement project. *Education + Training.* 2011;53(2/3):155–165.

24. Health Careers. *Health Careers.* Accessed September 25, 2023. https://www.healthcareers.nhs.uk/

25. Aberdeen T, Yin RK. (2009). *Case Study Research: Design and Methods* (4th Ed.). Sage. *CJAR.* 2013;14(1):69–71.

26. Baxter P, Jack S. Qualitative case study methodology: Study design and implementation for novice researchers. *The Qualitative Report.* Published online January 14, 2015. doi:10.46743/2160-3715/2008.1573

27. Cousin G *Researching Learning in Higher Education: An Introduction to Contemporary Methods and Approaches.* Routledge; 2009.

28. Kanuka H Characteristics of effective and sustainable teaching development programmes for quality teaching in higher education. *Higher Education Management.* 2010;22(2):1–14.
29. Mebert L, Barnes R, Dalley J, et al. Fostering student engagement through a real-world, collaborative project across disciplines and institutions. *Higher Education Pedagogies.* 2020;5(1):30–51.
30. Bandura A, Freeman WH, Lightsey R. Self-efficacy: The exercise of control. *Journal of Cognitive Psychotherapy.* 1999;13(2):158–166.
31. O'Keeffe P A sense of belonging: Improving student retention. *College Student Journal* 2013;47(4):605–613.
32. Cohen GL, Garcia J. Identity, belonging, and achievement: A model, interventions, implications. *Current Directions in Psychological Science.* 2008;17(6):365–369.
33. Lizzio A, Wilson K. Action learning in higher education: An investigation of its potential to develop professional capability. *Studies in Higher Education.* 2004;29(4):469–488.
34. Lave J *Cognition in Practice: Mind, Mathematics and Culture in Everyday Life.* Cambridge University Press; 1988.
35. Garrick J, Usher R. Flexible learning, contemporary work and enterprising selves. *Electronic Journal of Sociology.* 2000;5(1):1–15.
36. Kenyon C, Hase S. *Moving from Andragogy to Heutagogy in Vocational Education.* 2001.
37. Astin A. A look at pluralism in the contemporary student population. *NASPA Journal.* 1984;21(3):2–11.

11 Professional and career management

Developing employability and career skills for undergraduate and postgraduate biomedical science students

Georgina Larkin and Liz O'Gara

The changing landscape of the biomedical science job market

The biomedical science (BMS) job market has undergone significant transformations in recent years, driven by a variety of factors that include technological advancements, globalisation, and even unforeseen challenges such as the COVID-19 pandemic[1]. These changes have led to a diversification of career paths, moving beyond the traditional roles in laboratory research and healthcare settings. For instance, biomedical science graduates are now increasingly sought after in sectors such as data analytics, bioinformatics, pharmaceutical sales, and even science communication. This trend towards interdisciplinary collaboration has opened doors to roles that require a blend of skills, from both the scientific and the social sciences.

Alongside these new opportunities, the market has also become more competitive[2]. As technology advances, the skill set required of a biomedical scientist has expanded to include not just subject-specific knowledge but also proficiency in tools like machine learning algorithms or gene editing technologies like CRISPR. The globalisation of the job market also means that graduates often find themselves competing on an international stage, making adaptability and a broader skill set more crucial than ever.

Given the evolving nature of the biomedical science field, there is an urgent need to align the curriculum of biomedical science degrees with the skills that are actually in demand in the job market. Traditional curricula that focus solely on academic knowledge are increasingly seen as insufficient. Instead, a more holistic approach is advocated, one that combines rigorous academic training with a strong focus on career development and employability skills. Incorporating employability skills into the curriculum doesn't just mean teaching students how to write CVs or perform well in interviews, although those are important. It extends to fostering a set of transferable skills such as problem-solving, critical thinking, and effective communication, which are universally valued by employers[3]. Embedding career development into the curriculum involves guiding students through self-assessment and reflective learning, equipping them to make informed career choices. This is particularly crucial in a field as diverse and rapidly evolving as biomedical science.

DOI: 10.4324/9781003383994-16

Pedagogical models like DOTS[4] (decision learning, opportunity awareness, transition learning, self-awareness) and CareerEDGE[5,6] offer frameworks for achieving this integration. For example, they promote self-awareness, decision-making skills, and transitional learning, all key competencies for entering the job market. The biomedical science curriculum can be adapted to include modules or activities specifically aimed at career development, featuring real-world case studies, opportunities for internships or placements, and even mentoring programmes involving industry professionals. Modernising the biomedical science curriculum to focus on employability and career development is not just an educational imperative but also a socioeconomic one. As the field continues to evolve, so must the ways in which we prepare students to navigate this complex landscape. It is in the best interests of educational institutions, students, and the industry at large to invest in a curriculum that is both academically rigorous and professionally relevant.

In recent years, the biomedical science sector has seen a notable shift in recruitment trends[7], driven in part by the industry's response to emerging global challenges. For example, the COVID-19 pandemic has led to a surge in demand for professionals skilled in virology, immunology, and public health. Additionally, there is a growing focus on personalised medicine, which has led to increased recruitment in areas like genomics and bioinformatics. These trends are not just shaping the types of jobs available but are also influencing the qualifications and skills that employers are seeking. Soft skills such as adaptability, teamwork, and effective communication are now often considered as important as technical expertise. Further, interdisciplinary roles are emerging that require a blend of skills from both the biomedical sciences and other fields such as data science, ethics, and even business management.

Technological advancements have had a profound impact on the biomedical science sector, fundamentally altering the way research is conducted and care is delivered. Innovations in technologies like CRISPR for gene editing, AI for data analysis, and 3D printing for creating biological materials have created new avenues for research and treatment. These technologies are not just adding new dimensions to existing roles; they are creating entirely new job categories. For example, the rise of bioinformatics has led to a demand for professionals who are skilled both in biology and computer science.

Globalisation, too, has left an indelible mark. The ability to collaborate across borders has led to more international research partnerships, and the global harmonisation of regulatory standards is affecting everything from research protocols to product development. This internationalisation of the biomedical science sector means that graduates must now be prepared to work in a global context, which may require a wider range of skills including cultural competency and perhaps even multilingualism.

One of the most remarkable shifts in the biomedical science sector is the diversification of career paths available to graduates. Traditionally, careers in biomedical science were largely confined to research laboratories, healthcare settings, or academic institutions. While these avenues remain important, new opportunities have arisen in areas like consultancy, patent law relating to bio-medical inventions, science communication, and regulatory affairs. Some graduates are even leveraging their scientific background into entrepreneurial ventures, developing new biomedical products or services. Others are moving into policy roles, using their expertise to shape the healthcare policies of the future. These diversified career paths require a broader skill set than was previously needed, and they also offer the potential for a more varied and multidisciplinary professional life. This diversification is a double-edged sword though: while it offers more opportunities, it also demands that students are educated and trained in a way that prepares them for a wider array of potential career paths.

Navigating career development

Labour Market Information (LMI) is a useful tool for navigating career development. Information from a wide range of sources including university career services, academic mentors, recruitment platforms, and comprehensive graduate career websites all contributes to a holistic understanding of the opportunities and challenges in the biomedical science sector. This information provides a detailed overview of the current job market along with insights into various roles, requisite skill sets and potential career paths. Due to the evolving nature of biomedical science, accessing this type of information is essential for making well-informed career decisions. This goes beyond just choosing a job, it involves a deeper understanding of the professional development opportunities, work experience requirements and any additional qualifications that might enhance employability.

In the UK, various platforms provide LMI, for example Prospects[8], one of the most comprehensive graduate careers websites, outlines a wide range of roles and specialisations for biomedical science graduates. The importance of such information is magnified when considering the level of competition, especially for roles like Trainee Biomedical Scientists or Biomedical Scientists. The increasing number of students graduating from Institute of Biomedical Science (IBMS)-accredited degrees has intensified this competition, making it ever more important that students expand their career horizons and consider alternative routes, including emerging fields identified as shortage occupations by the UK Government[9].

Making sense of the network of career information needs strategic thinking and engagement from both academic institutions and students. Tools like the Career Readiness Survey (CRS)[10] have been instrumental in guiding curriculum planning and targeted career advice. The CRS is currently used by approximately 84 UK institutions and divides students into different stages of career planning. Each stage (decide, plan, compete, and sorted) represents a different level of readiness and presents its own set of challenges and requirements.

The decide stage groups those students who are still in the initial phases of their career decision-making process; they may not be sure of what they want to do or even what pathways are available. At the plan stage, students have generally identified their ideal career path but may lack a concrete strategy for getting there. The compete stage includes students who are well on their way to achieving their career goals but may need additional qualifications or experiences to help them stand out from the crowd. The sorted stage includes students who have a well-defined career path and are in the process of or have already secured a job or further education position. This categorisation allows academic and career advisors to offer tailored guidance, enhancing the relevance and effectiveness of their advice.

The fluid nature of career planning is also acknowledged through the CRS. Shifts can occur – those at the compete stage may find themselves back at the decide stage, perhaps due to a change in personal interest or market conditions. While surprising, these shifts offer important opportunities for reflection and course correction. Educators and career advisors can use these to reassess strategies, refocus efforts and if necessary, refine academic or skills development activities to better align with evolving career goals.

Pedagogical models and theories

In the context of career development and employability, several pedagogical models have gained prominence for their effectiveness and comprehensive approaches. Among these, the DOTS[4] model and CareerEDGE[11] are particularly noteworthy.

DOTS

The DOTS model serves as a comprehensive framework for career education, offering a structured approach that addresses the multifaceted nature of career planning and development. Comprising four key components – Decision learning, Opportunity awareness, Transition learning, and Self-awareness – this model aims to equip students with the essential skills and knowledge they need to navigate the complexities of the modern job market.

Decision learning focuses on the cognitive processes involved in making career-related choices. It encourages students to engage in critical thinking and decision-making exercises. For example, students might be asked to evaluate various career paths based on criteria such as job satisfaction, earning potential, and alignment with personal values. Educators can support this by offering workshops or courses that delve into decision-making theories and methodologies, thereby equipping students with the tools to make informed career choices. Opportunity awareness, the second component, aims to broaden students' understanding of the myriad career paths available to them. This is particularly crucial in fields that are rapidly evolving or have a wide range of specialisations. Universities can facilitate this by organising career fairs, inviting guest speakers from diverse professional backgrounds, and providing resources that outline different career opportunities within a given field. For example, a biomedical science student might be exposed to career paths in research, clinical diagnostics, pharmaceuticals, and even science communication. Transition learning is geared towards preparing students for the practical aspects of moving from education into employment. This involves equipping them with a range of soft and hard skills, from CV writing and interview techniques to networking and negotiation skills. Transition learning also covers practical aspects like understanding employment contracts, workplace ethics, and the dynamics of professional environments. Universities can offer workshops, mentorship programmes, and even mock interviews to prepare students for this transition. Self-awareness, the final pillar of the DOTS model, emphasises the importance of introspection and self-assessment in career planning. It encourages students to evaluate their skills, interests, and values, often through psychometric tests, reflective exercises, or one-on-one counselling sessions. This component is foundational, as a deep understanding of oneself provides the basis for all subsequent career-related decisions. Universities can support this by offering self-assessment tools and counselling services that help students identify their strengths and weaknesses, as well as their career inclinations.

While this traditional DOTS model has been a cornerstone in career education, it is argued that it's no longer sufficient, and that it needs to expand to consider the complexities of the modern world, including technological advancements and global economic shifts[12]. These changes don't just affect the job market; they also have significant implications on a student's early life experiences, social attachments, and values. Hence, a more nuanced approach is called for, one that incorporates the changing dynamics both globally and locally. New DOTS introduces a four-stage learning process to do this: Sensing, Sifting, Focusing, and Understanding. These stages are built on the belief that career management is a complex and dynamic learning process that needs to evolve over time. Sensing involves gathering information, sifting organises this information, focusing brings it into a mental framework, and understanding develops critical awareness. This sequence not only sets the scene for a student's career journey but also infuses it with emotional and social contexts, portraying a career as a narrative. It also emphasises the importance of 'learning to learn'. In a rapidly changing environment, knowing how to adapt is crucial. It also acknowledges the interconnectedness of various life roles, such as worker, partner, and citizen, advocating for a broader and deeper understanding of 'careers work' to replace what we traditionally understand as career education and guidance.

The New DOTS model offers a nuanced approach that can be particularly beneficial for biomedical science students. Biomedical science is a field that is highly dynamic, influenced by rapid technological advancements and ethical considerations and traditional career paths are being reshaped, requiring students to be adaptable and multifaceted in their skill sets. The sensing aspect of New DOTS can be integrated into career education to help students become aware of the variety of opportunities that extend beyond academia and traditional lab research. This could range from roles in public policy and bioethics to entrepreneurial ventures and medical communication. The sifting and focusing elements are also crucial. Biomedical science is an interdisciplinary field, and students often need to sift through a wealth of information and opportunities. Helping them organise this information effectively allows them to focus on what truly aligns with their skills and interests. For example, a student interested in both neuroscience and data science might focus on computational neuroscience as a career path. The focusing stage would then involve developing a more specific skill set, perhaps through targeted coursework or research projects. Understanding, the final stage in the New DOTS model, can help biomedical science students develop critical awareness about their chosen paths. This involves not just understanding the scientific aspects but also the ethical, social, and economic implications of their work. For example, a student interested in genetic engineering would benefit from understanding the ethical debates surrounding gene editing technologies like CRISPR. This comprehensive understanding is essential for making sustainable career decisions.

The emphasis on learning to learn, a skill that is indispensable in a field as fast-paced as biomedical science is also helpful. Students must be prepared to continually update their knowledge and skills, making them more resilient in a competitive job market. This involves understanding that career paths are increasingly non-linear, requiring adaptability and a willingness to change directions when needed. New DOTS also stresses the importance of understanding the interconnectedness of various life roles. Biomedical scientists don't exist in a vacuum; they are also citizens, partners, and perhaps future parents. Balancing these roles requires a more holistic approach to career planning, one that considers not just job prospects but also personal values and lifestyle choices.

CareerEDGE

The CareerEDGE[11] model offers a robust framework for understanding graduate employability, incorporating not only traditional indicators like academic achievement and work experience but also delving into more nuanced factors. Developed with the aim of providing a comprehensive overview of what contributes to employability, the model emphasises career development learning, experience, and emotional intelligence as vital elements. These components serve as a foundational triad that informs a graduate's readiness for the job market. Career development learning, in this context, is not limited to obtaining information about job opportunities or creating a CV. Rather, it entails a deeper engagement with a student's own career aspirations and the development of skills needed for long-term success. This often involves a blend of formal education and informal learning experiences, aimed at fostering a proactive approach to career planning. Experience, the second pillar, is interpreted broadly to encompass a range of activities that expose students to real-world scenarios. This could include activities like volunteer work, or extracurricular activities. The key is the transference and application of skills and knowledge in practical settings, which not only bolsters a student's CV but also provides essential soft skills like teamwork, communication, and problem-solving.

Emotional intelligence, the third cornerstone, is perhaps one of the most innovative aspects of the CareerEDGE model. Recognising that emotional competencies like self-awareness, empathy, and stress management are as important as technical skills, the model integrates these. The ability to navigate interpersonal relationships and adapt to varying workplace cultures is often what sets apart highly employable graduates from their peers. Yet, what truly distinguishes the CareerEDGE model is its focus on the concept of 'edge' – those supplementary attributes that offer graduates a competitive advantage in the job market. This is where social and cultural capital comes into play. Social capital relates to the networks and relationships that individuals form, which can often open doors that are otherwise hard to unlock. Cultural capital, on the other hand, involves an understanding and appreciation of the norms, values, and unwritten rules that govern professional settings. These forms of capital are increasingly recognised as vital, yet often overlooked, aspects of employability.

The application of the CareerEDGE model to career education for biomedical science students can significantly enrich the traditional curricula. Biomedical science is a field that not only demands a strong grasp of complex scientific concepts but also requires a range of other skills and attributes that are often not addressed adequately in a purely academic setting.

The first element of CareerEDGE, career development learning, has immediate implications for biomedical science students. Beyond acquiring scientific knowledge, these students must also develop an understanding of the diverse career paths available to them, ranging from research and academia to healthcare management and pharmaceuticals. Incorporating career development learning into the curriculum can help students make informed decisions about specialisations, further studies, or entering the workforce directly after graduation. For instance, workshops on grant writing, ethics in biomedical research, or healthcare policy could supplement traditional lectures and laboratory work. Experience, as the model suggests, is crucial in shaping a well-rounded biomedical scientist. Biomedical science students can benefit greatly from placements in clinical laboratories, research institutions, or even pharmaceutical companies. Not only does this give them a real-world perspective on the application of their studies, but it also equips them with practical skills that are often not covered in academic programmes. This experience could be invaluable when they embark on their professional journeys, giving them a tangible edge over graduates who have only been exposed to theoretical knowledge.

Emotional intelligence is particularly important in biomedical science, where professionals often find themselves at the intersection of science and human health. The ability to understand and manage emotions, as well as those of others, can be particularly important in settings like healthcare, where empathy and interpersonal skills are as important as technical competencies.

Emotional intelligence can be cultivated through mentoring programmes, peer reviews, and even through the integration of humanities and ethics courses into the biomedical science curriculum.

The concept of 'edge' in the CareerEDGE model can be translated into the biomedical science context as the additional skills or attributes that make a graduate more employable. Given the interdisciplinary nature of biomedical science, students who possess social and cultural capital may find it easier to navigate complex, multi-disciplinary teams, be it in research or clinical settings. Networking events, collaborations with industry, and international exchange programmes can all contribute to building this form of capital.

Career development through a biomedical science degree course

Pre-entry

Even before starting an academic journey, prospective students can begin to think about their career planning, particularly for fields like biomedical science where graduation doesn't necessarily end in a predetermined role in the NHS. University open days and applicant days are important events for starting these thinking processes. They can be designed to provide a comprehensive preview of the academic and career pathways that a degree can lead into.

We can also start students thinking about Continuing Professional Development (CPD) at these preliminary stages too. CPD is a lifelong commitment to skills development and can be useful for shaping and managing career aspirations[13]. If we introduce students to CPD early on, it can help them view their educational journey as one component of a larger, ongoing process of professional development. This can broaden their understanding of what a biomedical science degree can offer as well as manage their expectations realistically, potentially leading to reduced attrition rates.

First year

The first year of a biomedical science degree is a formative period that sets the stage for both academic and professional development. While the focus is often on foundational courses that provide a broad overview of the field, it's also an opportune time to begin the process of career planning. The initial year serves as an exploratory phase where students can start identifying their interests, strengths, and career aspirations within biomedical science and related fields.

One of the first steps in career planning at this stage is to engage in self-assessment and reflective learning. Students can benefit from taking stock of their skills and interests, often facilitated by career services through psychometric tests or one-on-one counselling. This self-awareness can guide students in making informed choices about their course, research opportunities, and even extracurricular activities that align with their career goals. Universities can support this by offering workshops or seminars that help students understand the diverse career paths available in biomedical science, from research and clinical practice to roles in healthcare management, policy, or medical writing.

Extracurricular involvement is another key aspect of career planning in the first year. Students are encouraged to join societies related to biomedical science or healthcare. These platforms offer networking opportunities and provide insights into various career paths. For example, a student who joins a biomedical research club may have the opportunity to hear guest lectures from professionals in the field, gaining a clearer understanding of what a career in biomedical research entails. Universities can facilitate this by providing information on relevant organisations and hosting events where students can interact with professionals and alumni.

While work placements are often more common in the later years of a degree, proactive students can start seeking out shadowing opportunities or even volunteer positions in healthcare settings. These experiences, although less intensive than formal placements, provide valuable exposure to the professional world and can help students make more informed career decisions. Universities can support this initiative by offering databases of volunteer opportunities and even credit-bearing community engagement programmes.

Academic networking should also not be overlooked in the first year. Building relationships with staff, peers and their academic advisors can open doors to research opportunities and provide valuable career advice.

First-year checklist

- Signpost to university career service, students' union, professional bodies' websites.
  - Encourage involvement in university life – societies, course-related events, attend career fairs and events, student course representative, student ambassador.
- Share your own career pathway and stories.
  - Encourage experiential learning such as volunteering, part-time work, internships.
- Link second-year module choices with specific career paths, where appropriate.
  - Promote professional development and career learning opportunities.

Second year
The second year of a biomedical science degree marks a significant transition for students, as they move from foundational courses to more specialised subjects that align closely with their career interests. This period is crucial for career planning, as students begin to gain a clearer understanding of the various pathways within biomedical science.

During this year, students often find it beneficial to engage more deeply with their academic advisors and career services. These interactions can help students refine their career goals and identify the skills and experiences they need to achieve them. Academic advisors can offer guidance on activities that students may benefit from in order to be well-prepared for their chosen career paths. For example, a student interested in genetic research might be advised to learn more about molecular biology and bioinformatics. Career services can provide additional support by offering workshops on CV writing, interview techniques, and job search strategies tailored to the biomedical sector.

Work-based learning opportunities become increasingly important at this stage. Placements and part-time jobs in relevant settings can offer invaluable practical experience. These experiences not only allow students to apply theoretical knowledge in real-world situations but also provide insights into the day-to-day workings of their chosen fields. For example, a student who secures a placement in a clinical laboratory will gain hands-on experience in diagnostic techniques, potentially confirming their interest in a career in clinical diagnostics. Work-based learning experiences are also not just opportunities for skill development but also potential launching pads for full-time employment. Many organisations use these programmes as a recruitment tool, offering high-performing students the chance to transition into permanent roles upon graduation. Therefore, excelling in these settings and building strong professional relationships can significantly impact a student's immediate career prospects. Universities can support this by offering career mentorship programmes, where students are paired with alumni or other professionals in their chosen fields for guidance and networking opportunities.

Networking also takes on greater importance in the second year. Students should be encouraged to attend industry conferences, engage with guest lecturers, and even seek informational interviews with professionals in their areas of interest. Many biomedical science-related professional societies offer student memberships, which can provide access to journals, networking events, and job listings. These memberships not only offer valuable resources but also demonstrate a level of professional commitment that can be appealing to future employers.

The skills and competencies gained during this year extend beyond technical expertise. Soft skills such as teamwork, communication, and problem-solving are often honed during group projects, presentations, and work placements. These skills are highly valued in the workplace and can significantly enhance a student's employability.

Second-year checklist

- Signpost to university career service, students' union, professional bodies' websites
  - Encourage attendance at career fairs and events.

- Invite course alumni into module and career sessions for short talks and networking opportunities.

  - Encourage more focused experiential learning such as volunteering (healthcare), part-time work, summer internships, year-long placements, day-a-week placements.

- Deadlines for graduate programmes and postgraduate study deadlines early in final year – especially for Medicine and Dentistry where external exams may be held over the summer.

  - Promote professional development and career learning opportunities.

- Suggest career guidance to students who are unclear about their career options.

Final year

The final year of a biomedical science degree is a critical juncture in a student's academic journey, serving as the gateway to their professional life. It's a period marked by a heightened focus on specialisation, whether that's in research, clinical practice, pharmaceuticals, or another subdiscipline within biomedical science. As students navigate this year, career planning takes on an urgency, requiring them to combine their academic experiences, practical skills, and professional aspirations into a coherent and actionable plan.

One of the first tasks in this final year should be to seek career guidance from both academic advisors and career services. At this stage, the guidance becomes more nuanced, often focusing on the specific steps needed to enter a chosen field. For example, students aiming for a research career might discuss the process of applying for PhDs, including the requirements of crafting a research proposal or preparing for subject-specific interviews. Career services can offer advanced workshops on job search strategies, tailoring CVs and cover letters for specific roles, and mastering interview techniques relevant to the biomedical sector.

Networking remains important, but the focus should now shift towards more targeted and strategic connections. Students can again be encouraged to attend conferences and also to engage with potential employers through social media platforms like LinkedIn.

The final year is also the time to consolidate and showcase the skills and competencies acquired throughout the degree. Students often find themselves involved in capstone projects that allow them to demonstrate their technical expertise, research skills, and soft skills like communication and teamwork. These projects not only serve as academic milestones but also as portfolio pieces that can be presented to potential employers.

Many graduate programmes and some forms of postgraduate study will open to applications at the start of the final year, so it is important that students are made aware of these opportunities to ensure they are ready to apply if they want to. Medicine, Dentistry and PGCE applications open in semester one for students to start the following year. Work with your career service to offer application support sessions to those students who are ready to apply for graduate opportunities at the beginning of their third year. The earlier the applications open, often the longer and more complicated the recruitment process is likely to be. Students need to be prepared for a range of recruitment activities, from online psychometric and personality tests to group exercises in assessment centres and multiple mini-interviews. Inviting employers or your career service to offer mock or practice sessions can boost confidence and improve results significantly. These sessions are more likely to fall into co- or extra-curricular activities as they will apply to a minority of students.

For institutions that use the CRS and related data, students can be easily identified at the start of their final year and strategies put in place to support their different stages of career readiness. We need to ensure those at the compete/sorted stages are supported with knowledge of deadlines and application processes. Those at the plan stage will often start looking for work in semester two, as peer and parental pressure starts to grow about what happens next. By this point, many students will have an idea of the general direction they want to go but may need some guidance on how to get there. There will also be a cohort who have an idea of what they want to do but choose to focus on their degree to achieve the best possible grade before they start to search and apply for jobs. Those at the decide stage may have no idea of what career path they want to take and may choose not to think about it at all until all undergraduate study is completed. This cohort will be more dependent on graduate support. It is widely recognised that this cohort is less likely to have engaged with extra-curricular career and employability activities as they do not consider them relevant to them. They may, in that case, be less likely to be aware of any ongoing graduate support offered. Unless students have engaged with career and employability teams during their undergraduate degree, they are more likely to seek the advice of their academic staff. Dissertation and final year project supervisors can play a part here by making students aware of support and signposting them appropriately.

For all students in their final year, anxiety about the future is likely to be increased with the pressure of final year projects or dissertations, final year modules and uncertainty about the future. This, together with peer and parental pressure can cause increased anxiety about what happens after graduation. For some career choices, the final degree classification can heavily influence the next decisions. If a first or 2:1 is required but not achieved, then a plan B may be necessary. A backup plan can be useful for all students with a firm idea of what they want to do, in case they are not successful immediately. Often, a few months or a year of work experience post-graduation can result in more successful applications to jobs and training programmes.

Final-year checklist

- Signpost to graduate schemes and relevant deadlines from induction/ Semester 1

  - Suggest career guidance to students who are unclear about their career options.

- Signpost to application support.

  - Advise on how to obtain academic references.

- Share the above information with academic advisor/final-year project supervisors.

  - Advise on opportunities and limitations of using artificial intelligence for job applications

- Signpost to graduate support and alumni networks

Masters level

Embarking on a masters course represents a significant step in academic and professional development, often serving as a bridge between foundational undergraduate studies and either specialised employment or further academic research. Career planning during a masters course is a nuanced process that requires a strategic approach, given the shorter duration of the programme and its specialised nature.

One of the first steps in career planning at this level involves a detailed consultation with academic advisors and career services. These consultations are more specialised than those at the undergraduate level, focusing on the unique demands and opportunities within the student's chosen field. For instance, a masters student specialising in biomedical data science would receive guidance on the specific skills and certifications that are most valued in that sector, such as proficiency in machine learning algorithms or data analytics tools.

Research projects take on a heightened importance during a masters course. Given the specialised nature of these programmes, such experiences are often directly aligned with career goals and provide an opportunity to gain advanced skills and knowledge. For example, a masters student in public health might undertake a project evaluating healthcare policies, gaining not only research skills but also insights into policy analysis that will be directly applicable to their future career. This work not only demonstrates technical skills but also soft skills like project management, problem-solving, and written communication, which are highly valued in the job market.

Networking remains important at masters level. As well as encouraging students to attend conferences and seminars, they may also pursue publication of their research to gain visibility in their field.

Masters checklist

- Begin searching graduate schemes in field of interest.
- Encourage students to discuss their options with career services.
- Integrate university support for CV writing, cover letter writing, interview technique etc into professional development modules/sessions.
- Ensure students know who would be a suitable academic referee.

International students

In the 20/21 academic year, international students made up approximately 22% of the total student population, 15.7% of the undergraduate population and 39.1% of the postgraduate population[14]. This international cohort brings with it a wide range of experiences and challenges, one of which is often a lack of work experience, which is further complicated by the cultural adjustments necessary for transitioning to a new country.

The importance of work experience in employability cannot be overstated. According to the Employer Perspectives Survey (EPS)[15], 65% of employers in the UK deemed relevant work experience an important factor in their recruitment decisions. A more recent survey by the Institute of Student Employers (ISE)[16] also emphasised that work experience significantly improved candidate's performance in the recruitment process, particularly when competence-based techniques were used. However, international students often encounter hurdles when trying to secure paid work experience in the UK due to visa restrictions[17]. One initial strategy to try and mitigate these hurdles is for universities to partner with local businesses to create work placement opportunities specifically tailored for international students. Another avenue worth exploring is the provision of virtual placements, these could also provide students with a chance to gain UK work experience even before they start their course. It's worth considering having a dedicated international students branch to central career services as well. Such a branch could offer workshops on writing CVs tailored to UK employers, understanding the UK work culture or guidance on job searching in the UK. It may also be possible to set up mentorship programmes that pair international students with alumni who have already successfully navigated the UK job market.

International students' checklist

- Ensure students are informed about visa options.
  - Signpost to Graduate Visa[18].
- Offer workshops related to working in the UK.
- Connect students with international alumni already working in the UK.

Student and graduate challenges

Understanding the complex challenges that students and graduates face enables academic staff to support students to develop the attributes that they need to complete in today's job market. These challenges are summarised in Tomlinson's Graduate Capital Model[19]:

- Human capital: Both the subject-specific and transferrable skills students need in their careers.
- Social capital: Networks, relationships, and social norms.
- Cultural capital: Understanding and appreciation of the distinct cultures that exist within sectors.
- Psychological capital: An individual's resilience, optimism, self-efficacy, and adaptability.
- Identity capital: Cumulative effect of an individual's experiences, values, and accomplishments that shape their professional profile.

Students lacking in these areas may face a series of challenges when entering the workplace, for example, students from less privileged backgrounds may not have the luxury of unpaid placements or extra-curricular activities and so may limit their exposure to practical skills and industry-specific knowledge. Such deficits can result in lower employability, making it harder for these students to compete in job interviews or even identify career paths. This can further exacerbate social inequality, reinforcing a cycle of limited opportunities and inhibited career development.

Addressing any deficits in these areas requires concerted efforts from universities, industry stakeholders, and policymakers alike. Strategies for mitigating these gaps can include mentorship programmes that pair students with professionals in their field of interest. Universities could also offer workshops on networking skills, CV writing, and interview techniques, specifically targeting students who might not have access to this kind of guidance at home. Financial support in the form of scholarships for networking events or industry conferences can also be instrumental in levelling the playing field. Fostering a campus culture that values diversity and inclusion can also go a long way in empowering all students, regardless of their capital.

Recommendations

Embedding career development and employability within the biomedical science curriculum is an imperative that goes beyond academic instruction. It aims to equip students with the skills, knowledge, and networks they need to thrive in an increasingly competitive job market. Key recommendations for achieving this include the integration of industry-relevant modules that focus on real-world applications of biomedical science. These could range from data analytics in healthcare to pharmaceutical development, thereby providing a comprehensive understanding of the field's scope. Another recommendation is the incorporation of soft skills training, such as communication, teamwork, and ethical considerations, which are often as crucial as technical skills in professional settings.

Work placements could also be a part of the curriculum. These experiences offer students invaluable insights into the workings of the industry and can often lead to job offers post-graduation. Mentorship programmes that connect students with professionals in the field can also provide tailored career advice and open doors to networking opportunities. Finally, a focus on interdisciplinary learning, which could involve modules in business management or ethics, can provide a well-rounded education that prepares students for various career paths, including entrepreneurship and research.

Looking towards future directions for research and practice, there is a need for longitudinal studies that assess the long-term impact of embedding career development and employability in the biomedical science curriculum. Such research could provide data-driven insights into the efficacy of different approaches, feeding into informing curriculum design. Also, as the field of biomedical sciences is ever-evolving, continuous curriculum updates are essential to keep pace with industry advancements. This could involve partnerships with industry stakeholders to ensure that the curriculum remains relevant and up-to-date.

In terms of practice, there is a growing need for a focus on digital literacy, given the increasing role of technology in healthcare. Future curricula should, therefore, include modules on digital healthcare solutions, data privacy, and cybersecurity. As the global landscape becomes more interconnected, an emphasis on international perspectives and cultural competency will become increasingly important as well.

Case study: An integrated approach to career development in biomedical science

A fundamental aspect of all degrees, not just biomedical science is the integration of career development skills, ideally at every level. Central to this is the inclusion of professional skills and career development-focused modules. In each year, students undertake these modules, tailored to the developmental milestones expected at that particular level of study. The inclusion of these modules should be combined with the involvement of central career services who provide input into their content and assessment. This can be further supported by the provision of bespoke events designed to further increase the employability of our students, for example training sessions focused on becoming a Physician's Associate, Clinical Scientist or even industry-sponsored lab sessions.

First year: Practical and study skills

In the first year, the study skills module is designed to be both practical and focused, offering students a toolkit that's directly applicable to their academic and professional lives. The module begins by teaching basic but essential skills and aims to support students in becoming self-sufficient learners. It helps them to identify their individual learning styles and needs, encouraging them to be proactive in their educational journey. The overall goal is to train students to think critically about their learning process, something they'll need to do throughout their careers.

Intended learning objectives:

1 To develop group working, communication, and problem-solving skills, mimicking the collaborative nature of most biomedical settings.
2 To provide a well-rounded set of study skills that will aid students in diverse academic tasks.
3 To ensure competence in key technical areas like numeracy, IT, data handling, scientific writing, and information retrieval.
4 To introduce students to laboratory practices, offering them basic competencies that will be required in more advanced courses and eventually in professional settings.

Second year: Professional and scientific practice

In the second-year module, attention shifts from basic academic preparation to skill sets that directly align with professional needs. It blends practical competencies with an understanding of the professional landscape in biomedical science. The module teaches more than advanced numeracy and laboratory skills. It also includes instrument calibration, data recording and trailing, as well as related health and safety documentation. These are elements that students are likely to encounter in a professional biomedical setting and mastering them will make them more attractive candidates for employment. The module goes further by integrating content that fosters a sense of professional identity. It discusses the roles of professional bodies such as the IBMS and the Royal Society of Biology (RSB), outlining their significance in career development. It also covers the importance of ISO accreditation, GLP (Good Laboratory Practice), and GMP (Good Manufacturing Practice), which are benchmarks for quality in scientific work. Bioethical considerations are also included, acknowledging the ethical complexities often faced in biomedical professions.

Intended learning objectives:

1 Plan and manage a laboratory project, including submission of Health & Safety and COSHH documentation.
2 Explain the importance of quality control and quality assurance and their role in good lab practice.
3 Analyse the ethical issues that arise in good lab practice.
4 Demonstrate knowledge of what employability means to an employer.

Final year: Enterprise in Biomedical Science

In the final year the emphasis of skills development moves to the application of these competencies in real-world scenarios. This module has a dual focus:

one is to deepen subject matter expertise, and the other is to cultivate a business-oriented perspective on biomedical science.

An important aspect of this module is its introduction of commercialisation and enterprise in the realm of biomedical science. Students are taught to understand how scientific discoveries and medical technologies can be taken from the lab bench to the marketplace. Students are also encouraged to understand and experience teamwork in a more nuanced manner. Unlike earlier modules that may focus simply on 'working well with others,' this takes a deep dive into the roles within teams and how effective collaboration can drive project success, especially in complex fields. The module also includes a self-reflection assessment, requiring students to articulate the transferable skills they have developed. This serves as a key experience, providing students with the opportunity to consolidate their learning journey and to understand how their skills can be applied in various professional contexts. By the end of this module students are well-versed in the business and teamwork skills that will make them effective professionals, contributing to the development of industry-ready professionals who can navigate both the scientific and commercial landscapes of biomedical science.

Intended learning objectives

1 To grasp the process of taking new ideas in biomedical science from concept to commercial reality.
2 To gather and organise both research and commercial information related to a specific biomedical science topic.
3 To critically evaluate their own group working skills and reflect on the importance of effective teamwork.
4 To synthesise the gathered information into a well-reasoned business model, executive summary, and presentation.

Masters level: Professional development

At masters level, there is a need for a more focused approach to career development and this module underscores this by targeting advanced skills like project management and leadership. Unlike undergraduate modules that may focus on foundational or transferable skills, this module addresses capabilities that are often immediately applicable in high-stakes, professional environments. Students are prompted to critically evaluate and reflect on their skills, allowing them to identify gaps and needs in their career development. The module assessment includes the production of a functioning career plan. This is an actionable roadmap that aligns a student's academic and professional skills with real-world opportunities and is designed to guide them in navigating their imminent transition from academic to professional life.

By the end of the module, students are expected to have a comprehensive understanding of how to manage complex projects and lead teams effectively.

They are also equipped with the reflective tools to continuously assess and adapt their skill sets and career plans as they progress in their fields. In essence, this module aims to produce individuals who are not only experts in their respective fields but also skilled managers and thoughtful, evolving professionals.

Intended learning objectives

1 To cultivate an understanding of project management and leadership skills and recognise their relevance in a research or professional setting.
2 To use critical reflection as a tool for informed and reasoned professional decision-making.
3 To examine one's research or practice methods critically, with a view to identifying what future learning may be needed to achieve career goals.
4 To engage in evaluation and analysis of one's project management skills, allowing targeted development in this area.

Conclusion

The biomedical science job market has experienced profound changes in recent years, marked by technological advancements, globalisation, and significant societal shifts such as those brought about by the COVID-19 pandemic. These developments have not only diversified the career paths available to graduates but also intensified competition in the field. Consequently, there is a pressing need to reform biomedical science curricula to better align with the evolving demands of the job market. This involves a shift from a purely academic focus to a more holistic approach that incorporates employability skills and career development.

For students, navigating this changing job market requires a proactive approach to career development. This entails using resources like LMI, engaging in work placements, and developing a broad skill set that includes both technical expertise and soft skills like adaptability and effective communication. Networking and building professional relationships are also crucial for success in this competitive field. The DOTS and CareerEDGE models provide valuable frameworks for integrating career education into the biomedical science curriculum. These models emphasise the development of decision-making skills, opportunity awareness, self-awareness, and the ability to navigate transitions, as well as the importance of experience, emotional intelligence, and the 'edge' factors like social and cultural capital. In practice, this means embedding modules and activities that focus on professional skills, ethical considerations, and industry awareness alongside traditional academic content.

Ultimately, preparing for a career in biomedical science in today's world requires more than just academic excellence. It demands a comprehensive understanding of the industry, a versatile skill set, and a strategic approach to career planning. The integration of career development into the biomedical science curriculum is not merely an academic necessity but a critical step in ensuring that graduates are equipped to thrive in a diverse and ever-evolving job market.

References

1. Bosch G, Casadevall A. Graduate biomedical science education needs a new philosophy. *MBio*. 2017;8(6). doi:10.1128/mBio.01539-17
2. Ghaffarzadegan N, Hawley J, Larson R, Xue Y. A note on PhD population growth in biomedical sciences. *Systems Research and Behavioral Science*. 2015;23(3):402–405.
3. McGunagle D, Zizka L. Employability skills for 21st-century STEM students: The employers' perspective. *Higher Education, Skills and Work-Based Learning*. 2020;10(3):591–606.
4. Law B, Watts AG. The dots analysis. *National Institute for Careers Education and Counselling, The Career-Learning NETWORK*. Published online 2003. http://www.hihohiho.com/memory/cafdots.pdf
5. Dacre-Pool L Revisiting the CareerEDGE model of graduate employability. *Journal of the National Institute for Career Education and Counselling*. 2020;44(1):51–56.
6. Dacre Pool L, Sewell P. The CareerEDGE model of graduate employability. *Pedagogy for employability 2012, implications for*. Published online 2012. https://scholar.google.ca/scholar?cluster=764099730764813985&hl=en&as_sdt=0,5&sciodt=0,5
7. Xu H, Gilliam RST, Peddada SD, Buchold GM, Collins TRL. Visualizing detailed postdoctoral employment trends using a new career outcome taxonomy. *Nature Biotechnology*. 2018;36(2):197–202.
8. Prospects.ac.uk. Accessed October 17, 2023. https://www.prospects.ac.uk/
9. Migration Advisory Committee. *A Guide to the Shortage Occupation List (SOL)*. Migration Advisory Committee; 2020.
10. The Association of Graduate Careers Advisory Services. *First-Year Student Career Readiness Report 2018*; 2018.
11. Pool LD, Sewell P. The CareerEDGE model of graduate employability. *Retrieved from C: UsersInnocentDownloadsTWO63*. Published online 2007.
12. Law B *New DOTS: Career Learning for the Contemporary World*. NICEC; 2001.
13. Alsop A *Continuing Professional Development in Health and Social Care: Strategies for Lifelong Learning*. John Wiley & Sons; 2013.
14. HESA. Higher Education Student Statistics: UK, 2021/22 - Where students come from and go to study. Accessed October 17, 2023. https://www.hesa.ac.uk/news/19-01-2023/sb265-higher-education-student-statistics/location
15. Shury J, Vivian D, Spreadbury K, et al. Employer Perspectives Survey 2014: Technical Report. Published 2014. Accessed October 17, 2023. http://doc.ukdataservice.ac.uk/doc/7614/mrdoc/pdf/7614_eps2014_technical_report.pdf
16. Institute of Student Employers. *Inside Student Recruitment*. Institute of Student Employers; 2019.
17. Student visa. Gov.uk. Published January 29, 2014. Accessed October 16, 2023. https://www.gov.uk/student-visa
18. Graduate visa. Gov.uk. Published July 1, 2021. Accessed October 16, 2023. https://www.gov.uk/graduate-visa
19. Graduate Capital Model. Accessed October 17, 2023. https://www.southampton.ac.uk/careers/staff/employability-exchange/index.page

Afterword

In this afterword, we take a moment to reflect on and consolidate the array of themes and insights presented in this text, focusing on the multifaceted aspects of biomedical science education. Our journey through these chapters has spanned various critical elements, from the intricacies of curriculum design to the broader implications of wide-ranging educational strategies on future professionals and the field at large.

We have explored the nuances involved in constructing a curriculum that is not only academically rigorous but also deeply attuned to the practical realities of the biomedical field. We have considered how a well-crafted curriculum must evolve continuously, keeping pace with the rapid advancements in scientific research and the changing landscape of healthcare. This evolution is about keeping the curriculum alive and responsive and in tune with the latest advancements. Such an approach to curriculum design and delivery produces a course that develops graduates who are not only knowledgeable in their field but also capable of applying their knowledge in diverse and often challenging environments. We can support the development of professionals who are adaptable, ethical, and equipped to contribute meaningfully to the biomedical field, whether in research, clinical settings, or industry.

Looking ahead, the trajectory of biomedical science education is set to be deeply influenced by the capacity to adapt and respond to the fluid landscape of science and healthcare. Biomedical science is inherently fast-paced and subject to continuous change, driven by rapid advancements in numerous areas. The future of education in this field, therefore, lies in its ability to keep pace with these changes and proactively incorporate them into the curriculum.

The advancements in biomedical technology are particularly significant. Breakthroughs in areas such as genomics, personalised medicine, biotechnology, and data analytics are revolutionising our understanding of health and disease. These advancements are not just theoretical; they have practical implications for many aspects of disease diagnosis, treatment, and prevention and as such, the biomedical science education must evolve to include them, ensuring that students are well-versed in the latest scientific advancements and also proficient in applying them in a professional context. Similarly, shifts in healthcare practices, especially within systems like the NHS, play a critical role in shaping

DOI: 10.4324/9781003383994-17

the future of biomedical science education. Changes in patient care models, the integration of new diagnostic tools, and evolving healthcare policies must be reflected in the curriculum. This ensures that graduates are not only prepared to work within these systems but can also contribute to their evolution and improvement.

Broader societal needs must also continually inform the development of biomedical science education. As global health challenges evolve, so too must the educational focus. This may involve a greater emphasis on emerging public health concerns, environmental impacts on health, or the ethical considerations of new medical technologies, and by staying attuned to these societal shifts, biomedical science education will remain relevant and vital to addressing current and future health challenges.

In essence, the future of biomedical science education is contingent upon its flexibility and foresight. A curriculum that is current and forward-looking and that anticipates and responds to the rapid changes in science and healthcare is essential for preparing students to excel in this field. By taking this approach, we equip our students not just with knowledge and skills, but with the adaptability and innovation mindset necessary to lead and thrive in their chosen career path, being well-equipped to contribute effectively in a global, interconnected world, addressing complex health challenges with innovative, multidisciplinary solutions. This approach to education is not just beneficial but essential for the advancement of biomedical science and for addressing the health needs of societies around the world. As educators, our role is to facilitate this process, ensuring that the education we provide remains at the cutting edge of both scientific advancement and educational excellence. By doing so, we not only uphold the standards of the discipline but also contribute to shaping a future workforce that is equipped to tackle the health challenges of tomorrow. Our collective efforts in this endeavour will not only benefit our students but also contribute significantly to the advancement of biomedical science and the betterment of global health and well-being.

Index

Pages in **bold** refer to tables.

For Product Safety Concerns and Information please contact our EU
representative GPSR@taylorandfrancis.com
Taylor & Francis Verlag GmbH, Kaufingerstraße 24, 80331 München, Germany